...IG THERAPY SERIES

Relationship Counselling:
Sons and Their Mothers

A Person-Centred Dialogue

Richard Bryant-Jefferies

Radcliffe Publishing
Oxford • San Francisco

Radcliffe Publishing Ltd
18 Marcham Road
Abingdon
Oxon OX14 1AA
United Kingdom

www.radcliffe-oxford.com
Electronic catalogue and worldwide online ordering facility.

© 2004 Richard Bryant-Jefferies

British Library Cataloguing in Publication Data

A catalogue record for this book is available from the British Library.

ISBN 1 85775 648 7

Typeset by Aarontype Limited, Easton, Bristol
Printed and bound by TJ International Ltd, Padstow, Cornwall

Contents

Foreword

In his remarkable *Living Therapy* series Richard Bryant-Jefferies invented a new way of showing how counselling works. The fictitious dialogues of *Relationship Counselling: Sons and Their Mothers* offer a creative possibility for both counsellors and (potential) clients to deal with the practice and theory of counselling.

The book is indeed a person-centred dialogue in many ways. It includes not only a most interesting and exciting counselling dialogue, it also stimulates a dialogue between the reader and the book (and its counsellor, its client and its supervisor), and it may well serve as a basis for a dialogue among trainees and offer many opportunities for further training.

Relationship Counselling provides an interesting and inspiring approach for therapists to reflect on their practice. The narrative stimulates readers to consider their own approach to clients. By checking personal reactions to the way the counsellor in the book proceeds and to the story's unfolding process, the practitioner will find him- or herself reflecting on the similarities and differences to his or her own way of working. In dealing with the explanations given one's own theories are challenged and fostered to be further developed. Furthermore, the portrayal of the supervision sessions stimulates thinking about the various possibilities for making use of the supervisor–supervisee relationship, furthering consideration of possible alternatives to the counsellor's way of using this powerful tool to increase the facilitative potential of the persons involved in the counselling process. References to new developments and recent literature support the important ongoing personal theory development of the counsellor who makes use of the book for his or her reflections. Using the book and its discussion points to examine and consider personal and authentic alternatives in the single responses, as well as in the forming of the relationship as a whole, can be of considerable value in training and supervision.

On the other hand the narrative makes the practice of counselling available to people who are thinking of seeing a counsellor but who are not yet sure whether they should do so or what type of counselling relationship they seek. Reading this book will help give an impression of what person-centred counselling is about and how it can be used for oneself. The reader gains insight into the counselling relationship and how the counselling process may feel and look. Clients who already have counselling experience may feel stimulated to mull over their own experiences, insights and developments.

For persons interested in the person-centred approach this book serves as an easy-to-read introduction to the concept and method founded by Carl Rogers and continuously elaborated since. The book presents the state of the art of this approach to counselling and psychotherapy and Richard Bryant-Jefferies' descriptions show his thinking and working in up-to-date relational settings. In the last few decades the centrality of relationship in counselling and therapy has become important to almost all orientations and modalities. Within the person-centred world the importance and impact of the encounter between client and counsellor has become more and more acknowledged. Such a relationship-oriented understanding of person-centred work focuses equally on the intrapersonal and the interpersonal. The inner process in the client and the counsellor and the process between them are mutually related and important for the facilitation of the client's personality development and move towards autonomy and mature interrelatedness. Person-centred theoreticians and practitioners around the globe have become more and more aware that it is the acknowledgment of a common 'We' of our existence that builds the foundation for a facilitative relationship, and it is therefore the counsellor's presence that supports the client in their endeavour to become the person they want to be. It is the encounter, the relationship between the persons involved, that is the core of counselling, and it is respectful dialogue that constitutes the nature of the person-centred counselling process (Schmid, 2003). These aspects are clearly visible in the narrative of this book and the explanations and interpretations given. It not only clearly explains what is going on in both client and counsellor, it also reflects the relationship between them and between the supervisor and the counsellor.

Overall, this book is another example of the insight – as a genuine development from the foundations that Carl Rogers stated half a century ago – that the nature of counselling must be seen in the fact that 'it is the clients that make therapy work' (Bohart and Tallman, 1999; Bohart, 2004).

Peter F Schmid
Professor at the University of Graz, Austria
Faculty Member of Saybrook Graduate School, San Francisco
Founder of person-centred training in Austria
August 2004

References

Bohart AC (2004) How do clients make empathy work? *Person-Centered and Experiential Psychotherapies.* **3**(2): 102–17.

Bohart AC and Tallman K (eds) (1999) *How Clients Make Therapy Work.* American Psychological Association, Washington, DC.

Schmid PF (2003) The characteristics of a person-centered approach to therapy and counselling: Criteria for identity and coherence. *Person-Centered and Experiential Psychotherapies.* **2**(2): 104–20.

Preface

From the start of my own training in person-centred counselling the problematic potential of the mother–son relationship, and the under-emphasis on this within material written for counsellors, has struck me. How does a man break free from being 'son' and claim his independence as a male adult in his own right, and what difficulties can arise within this process? What happens when it does not occur, the son rendered effectively impotent as a man, being unable to psychologically free himself from the sense of being his mother's son?

From the opposite perspective, what happens when sons deliberately choose lifestyles that involve maintaining an identity as a dependent son, choosing a way of being that for whatever reason involves not taking responsibility and expecting to be bailed out by a mother who is caught in her own dependency trap? In such instances we see a mother being dragged down by the constant demands of a son who, in a certain sense, is unable, or unwilling, to grow up. Cycles of co-dependency develop. Mother and son sometimes caught in a dance which enables both to cling to identities that perhaps should have passed away long ago – the son not wishing to affirm his identity as an independent adult; the mother unwilling to let go of certain aspects of her self-concept or identity as 'mother' and create the space and the opportunity to embrace a fresh phase in her own life.

This latest volume of the *Living Therapy* series concentrates on one man (Peter) in his struggle to claim an independent lifestyle and resolve the effects of what he experienced as a rejecting and loveless childhood. From the time that he enters into therapy, the client finds himself on a journey towards a greater realisation of his need to move on, encountering past experiences that were major factors in his own conditioned development, and engaging in new experiences which contribute to a process of redefining himself and his potentialities.

Included in this volume is material to inform the training process of counsellors and many others who seek to work with people experiencing these relational dynamics. *Relationship Counselling: Sons and Their Mothers* is intended as much for experienced counsellors as it is for trainees. It provides real insight into what can occur during counselling sessions. I hope it will raise awareness of, and inform, not only person-centred practice within this relational context, but also contribute to other theoretical approaches within the world of counselling and psychotherapy. Reflections on the therapeutic process and points for discussion are included to stimulate further thought and debate.

Relationship Counselling: Sons and Their Mothers will also be of value to the many healthcare and social care professionals who, while they may specialise in other areas such as substance misuse, stress, family therapy or couple counselling, will find that the mother–son relationship has impact on the work they are doing. For all these professionals, the text contributes to demystifying what can occur in therapy, and at the same time provides useful ways of working that may be used by professionals other than counsellors.

I hope that this book contributes to developing further our understanding of the causes and the often painful and lasting impact of difficult mother–son relationships, as well as how to work with the person so affected who, in adulthood, realises that they are, as Peter (the client) describes it, 'caged up in myself by the rejection and lack of love that was inflicted on me'.

Richard Bryant-Jefferies
July 2004

About the author

Richard Bryant-Jefferies qualified as a person-centred counsellor/therapist in 1994 and remains passionate about the application and effectiveness of this approach. Between early 1995 and mid 2003 Richard worked at a community drug and alcohol service in Surrey, though more recently he has been appointed to manage NHS substance misuse services in the Royal Borough of Kensington and Chelsea in London, part of the Central and North West London Mental Health NHS Trust. He has experience of offering both counselling and supervision in NHS, GP and private settings, and has provided training through 'alcohol awareness and response' workshops.

Richard had his first book on a counselling theme published in 2001, *Counselling the Person Beyond the Alcohol Problem* (Jessica Kingsley Publishers), providing theoretical yet practical insights into the application of the person-centred approach within the context of the 'cycle of change' model that has been widely adopted to describe the process of change in the field of addiction. Since then he was been writing for the *Living Therapy* series (Radcliffe Medical Press), producing an ongoing series of person-centred dialogues: *Problem Drinking*, *Time Limited Therapy in Primary Care*, *Counselling a Survivor of Child Sexual Abuse*, *Counselling a Recovering Drug User*, *Counselling Young People* and *Counselling for Progressive Disability*. The aim of the series is to bring the reader a direct experience of the counselling process, an exposure to the thoughts and feelings of both client and counsellor as they encounter each other on the therapeutic journey, and an insight into the value and importance of supervision.

Richard is keen to bring the experience of the therapeutic process, from the standpoint and application of the person-centred approach, to a wider audience. He is convinced that the principles and attitudinal values of this approach and the emphasis it places on the therapeutic relationship are key to helping people create greater authenticity both in themselves and in their lives, leading to a fuller and more satisfying human experience.

Acknowledgements

Over the years I have listened to many different versions of the sons and mothers relationship – some problematic and challenging, others where there has remained a genuine mutual love and respect that has enabled healthy and mature adult-to-adult relationships to develop. Without doubt, this has contributed to my thoughts as I have been writing this latest volume in the *Living Therapy* series.

I am also grateful to Peter Schmid for his Foreword.

I would also like to thank, once again, the series editor, Maggie Pettifer, for her continued support, energy, enthusiasm and encouragement in the writing of the *Living Therapy* series.

Introduction

The aim of the *Living Therapy* series is to offer the reader an opportunity to experience and to appreciate, through the use of dialogue, some of the diverse and challenging issues that can arise during counselling (Bryant-Jefferies, 2003a, 2003b, 2004) – quite a unique approach in the wide world of counselling literature. Perhaps, now that the seventh book in this series has been written, this approach is not so unique! *Relationship Counselling: Sons and Their Mothers* addresses the experience of working with an adult man who is confronted with the reality of the effects of a rejecting relationship with his mother, in both past and present.

Relationship Counselling: Sons and Their Mothers is composed of fictitious dialogues between a client and his counsellor, and between the counsellor and his supervisor. Within the dialogues are woven the reflective thoughts and feelings of the client, the counsellor and the supervisor, along with boxed comments on the process and references to person-centred theory.

The book has been written with the aim of demonstrating the counsellor's application of the person-centred approach (PCA) – a theoretical approach to counselling that has, at its heart, the power of the relational experience to offer the client an experience through which greater potential for authentic living may emerge. The approach is widely used by counsellors working in the UK today: in a membership survey in 2001 by the British Association for Counselling and Psychotherapy, 35.6 per cent of those responding claimed to work to the person-centred approach, while 25.4 per cent identified themselves as psychodynamic practitioners.

The reader may find it takes a while to adjust to the dialogue format. Many of the responses offered by the counsellor, Michael, are reflections of what the client, Peter, has said. This is not to be read as conveying a simple repetition of the client's words. Rather, the counsellor seeks to voice empathic responses, often with a sense of 'checking out' that he is hearing accurately what the client is saying. The client says something; the counsellor then conveys that he has heard it, sometimes with the same words, sometimes including a sense of what he feels may be being communicated through the client's tone of voice, facial expression, or simply the atmosphere of the moment. The client is then enabled to confirm that he has been heard accurately, or correct the counsellor in his perception. The client may then explore more deeply what they have been saying or move on, in either case with a sense that they have been heard and warmly accepted. To draw this to the reader's attention, I have included some of the inner thoughts and feelings that are present within the individuals who form the narrative.

The supervision sessions are included to offer the reader insight into the nature of therapeutic supervision in the context of the counselling profession, a method of supervising that I term 'collaborative review'. For many trainee counsellors, the use of supervision can be something of a mystery, and it is hoped that this book will go a long way to unravelling this. In the supervision sessions I seek to demonstrate the application of the supervisory relationship. My intention is to show how supervision of the counsellor is very much a part of the therapeutic process enabling the counsellor to be authentically and empathically present whilst offering unconditional positive regard.

Many professions do not recognise the need for some form of personal and process supervision, and often what is offered is line management. However, counsellors are required to receive regular supervision in order to explore the dynamics of the relationship with the client, the impact of the work on the counsellor and on the client, to receive support, and to provide an opportunity for an experienced co-professional to monitor the supervisee's work in relation to ethical standards and codes of practice. The supervision sessions are included because they are an integral part of the therapeutic process. It is also hoped that they will help readers from other professions to recognise the value of some form of supportive and collaborative supervision in order to help them become more authentically present with their own clients.

I also favour an approach that is of a collaborative nature, which I describe as a process of 'collaborative review'. Merry (2002) describes what he terms 'collaborative inquiry' as a 'form of research or inquiry in which two people (the supervisor and the counsellor) collaborate or co-operate in an effort to understand what is going on within the counselling relationship and within the counsellor'. There are, of course, as many models of supervision as there are models of counselling. In this book the supervisor is seeking to apply the attitudinal qualities of the person-centred approach.

It is the norm for all professionals working in the healthcare and social care environment in this age of regulation to be formally accredited or registered and to work to their own professional organisation's code of ethics or practice. For instance, registered counselling practitioners with the British Association for Counselling and Psychotherapy are required to have regular supervision and continuing professional development to maintain registration. While professions other than counsellors will gain much from this book in their work with adults affected by problematic relational experiences in childhood, it is essential that they follow the standards, safeguards and ethical codes of their own professional organisation, and are appropriately trained and supervised to work with their clients.

All characters in this book are fictitious and are not intended to bear resemblance to any particular person or persons.

The person-centred approach

The person-centred approach (PCA) was formulated by Carl Rogers, and references are made to his ideas within the text of the book. However, it will be helpful for readers who are unfamiliar with this way of working to have an appreciation of its theoretical base.

Rogers proposed that certain conditions, when present within a therapeutic relationship, would enable the client to develop towards what he termed 'fuller functionality'. Over a number of years he refined these ideas, which he defined as 'the necessary and sufficient conditions for constructive personality change'. These he described as follows.

1 Two persons are in psychological contact.
2 The first, whom we shall term the client, is in a state of incongruence, being vulnerable or anxious.
3 The second person, whom we shall term the therapist, is congruent or integrated in the relationship.
4 The therapist experiences unconditional positive regard for the client.
5 The therapist experiences an empathic understanding of the client's internal frame of reference and endeavours to communicate this experience to the client.
6 The communication to the client of the therapist's empathic understanding and unconditional positive regard is to a minimal degree achieved. (Rogers, 1957, p. 96)

The first necessary and sufficient condition given for constructive personality change is that of 'two persons being in psychological contact'. However, although he later published this as simply 'contact' (Rogers, 1959) it is suggested (Wyatt and Sanders, 2002, p. 6) that this was actually written in 1953–54. They quote Rogers as defining contact in the following terms: 'Two persons are in psychological contact, or have the minimum essential relationship when each makes a perceived or subceived difference in the experiential field of the other' (Rogers, 1959, p. 207). A recent exploration of the nature of psychological contact from a person-centred perspective is given by Warner (2002).

Rogers defined empathy as meaning 'entering the private perceptual world of the other ... being sensitive, moment by moment, to the changing felt meanings which flow in this other person ... It means sensing meanings of which he or she is scarcely aware, but not trying to uncover totally unconscious feelings' (1980, p. 142). It is a very delicate process, and it provides, I believe, a foundation block. The counsellor's role is primarily to establish empathic rapport and communicate empathic understanding to the client.

Within this relationship the counsellor seeks to maintain an attitude of unconditional positive regard towards the client and all that they disclose. This is not 'agreeing with', it is simply warm acceptance. Rogers wrote, 'when the therapist is experiencing a positive, acceptant attitude towards whatever the client *is* at that moment, therapeutic movement or change is more likely to occur' (1980, p. 116). Mearns and Thorne suggest that 'unconditional positive regard is the label given to the fundamental attitude of the person-centred counsellor towards her client. The counsellor who holds this attitude deeply values the humanity of her client and is not deflected in that valuing by any particular client behaviours. The attitude manifests itself in the counsellor's consistent acceptance of and enduring warmth towards her client' (Mearns and Thorne, 1988, p. 59).

Last, but by no means least, is that state of being that Rogers referred to as congruence, but which has also been described in terms of 'realness', 'transparency', 'genuineness', 'authenticity'. Indeed Rogers wrote that '. . . genuineness, realness or congruence . . . this means that the therapist is openly being the feelings and attitudes that are flowing within at the moment . . . the term transparent catches the flavour of this condition'. Putting this into the therapeutic setting, we can say that 'congruence is the state of being of the counsellor when her outward responses to her client consistently match the inner feelings and sensations which she has in relation to her client' (Mearns and Thorne, 1999, p. 84).

I would suggest that any congruent expression by the counsellor of their feelings or reactions has to emerge through the process of being in therapeutic relationship with the client. It is a disciplined response and not an open door to endless self-disclosure. Congruent expression is perhaps most appropriate and therapeutically valuable where it is informed by the existence of an empathic understanding of the client's inner world, and is offered in a climate of a genuine warm acceptance towards the client.

PCA regards the relationship that we have with our clients, and the attitude that we hold within that relationship, to be key factors. In my experience, many adult psychological difficulties develop out of life-experiences that involve problematic, conditional or abusive relational experiences. This can be centred in childhood or later in life. What is important is that the individual is left, through relationships that have a negative conditioning effect, with a distorted perception of themselves and their potential as a person. I see many people who have learned from childhood experience beliefs such as 'I can never be good enough to be praised for what I have achieved; I never match my parents' expectations' or 'No one was ever there for me when I was hurting; perhaps I am unlovable'. The result is a loss of a positive sense of self, and the individual adapts to maintain the newly learned concept of self. This is then lived out, possibly throughout life, with the person seeking to satisfy what they have come to believe about themselves: being unable to achieve, feeling unable or undeserving to be loved, though perhaps in both cases maintaining a constant desperation to receive what they never had. Yet, perversely, they may then sabotage any possibility of gaining what they want in order to maintain the negatively conditioned sense of self and the sense of satisfaction that this gives them because they have developed such a strong identity with it.

Obviously, relationships with parents will be a major conditioning factor in the development of the child on the journey towards adulthood. We learn about ourselves through the reactions of those closest to us. Even when they may not be experienced as being close, their consistent presence means that our view of ourselves is shaped by the experiences we have and the meanings that we attribute to them. The child's first relationship is with his mother. Her response is contributing to the child's emerging structure of self. Clearly a rejecting response will have a huge impact and will set up a chain reaction of 'self-beliefs' in the child that will be very different from those that develop where empathy, love, warmth, honesty and trust are present. The child will be left with a damaged sense of self which will then find expression in a range of attitudes and behaviours that are perhaps more likely to be problematic and difficult. Having established a structure of self and a way of being that is rooted in a negative set of childhood, relational experience with the first key object of relationship, it may then take a therapeutic encounter later in life to unravel the damage and help them to free themselves from views that they have about themselves and relationships and the associated behaviours that have developed.

I mention above the word 'love'. It is an important word though not necessarily one used to describe therapeutic relationship. Patterson, however, gives a valuable definition of love as it applies to the person-centred therapeutic process. He writes, 'we define love as an attitude that is expressed through empathic understanding, respect and compassion, acceptance, and therapeutic genuineness, or honesty and openness towards others' (2000, p. 315). We all need love, but most of all we need it during our developmental period of life. The same author affirms that 'while love is important throughout life for the well-being of the individual, it is particularly important, indeed absolutely necessary, for the survival of the infant and for providing the basis for the normal psychological development of the individual' (Patterson, 2000, pp. 314–15).

It is my belief that by offering someone a non-judgemental, warm and accepting, and authentic relationship – in truth an experience of love (perhaps we need to speak more of therapeutic love) – then that person can grow into a fresh sense of self in which their potential as a person can become more fulfilled. Such an experience fosters an opportunity for the client to redefine themselves as they experience the presence of the therapist's congruence, empathy and unconditional positive regard. This process can take time. Often the personality change that is required to sustain a shift away from what have been termed 'conditions of worth' requires a lengthy period of therapeutic work, bearing in mind that the person may be struggling to unravel a sense of self that has been developed, sustained and reinforced for many decades of life.

The term 'conditions of worth' applies to the conditioning that is frequently present in childhood, and at other times in life, when a person experiences that their worth is conditional on their doing something, or behaving, in a certain way. This is usually to satisfy someone else's needs, and can be contrary to the client's own sense of what would be a satisfying experience. The values of others become a feature of the individual's structure of self. The person moves away from being true to themselves, learning instead to remain 'true' to their conditioned sense of worth. This state of being in the client is challenged by the person-centred therapist by offering them unconditional positive regard and warm acceptance. Such a therapist, by genuinely offering these therapeutic attitudes, provides the client with an opportunity to be exposed to what may be a new experience or one that in the past they have dismissed, preferring to stay with that which matches and therefore reinforces their conditioned sense of worth and sense of self. Unconditional positive regard and warm acceptance offered consistently over time can, and does, enable clients to begin to question their beliefs about themselves and to begin to build into their structure of self the capacity to see and experience themselves as being of value for who they are. It enables them to liberate themselves from the constraints of patterns of conditioning.

A crucial feature or factor in this process is the presence of what Rogers termed 'the actualizing tendency', a tendency towards fuller and more complete personhood with an associated greater fulfilment of their potentialities. The role of the person-centred counsellor is to provide the facilitative climate within which this tendency can work constructively. 'The therapist trusts the actualizing tendency of the client and truly believes that the client who experiences the freedom of a fostering psychological climate will resolve his or her own problems' (Bozarth, 1998, p. 4). This is fundamental to the application of the person-centred approach. Rogers (1986, p. 198) wrote: 'the person-centred approach is built on a basic trust in the person . . . (It) depends on the actualizing tendency present in every living organism – the tendency to grow, to develop, to realize its full potential. This way of being trusts the constructive directional flow of the human being towards a more complex and complete development. It is this directional flow that we aim to release.'

The therapeutic relationship is central. A therapeutic approach such as person-centred affirms that it is not what you do so much as 'how you are' with your client that is therapeutically significant, and this 'how you are' has to be received by the client. Gaylin (2001, p. 103) highlights the importance of client perception. 'If clients believe that their therapist is working on their behalf – if they perceive caring and understanding – then therapy is likely to be successful. It is the condition of attachment and the perception of connection that have the power to release the faltered actualization of the self.' He goes on to stress how 'we all need to feel connected, prized – loved', describing human beings as 'a species born into mutual interdependence', and that there 'can be no self outside the context of others'. He highlights that 'loneliness is dehumanizing and isolation anathema to the human condition. The relationship' he suggests 'is what psychotherapy is all about.' Without doubt, and it seems too obvious to state it, the reaction of a parent to a child – and in the case of this book, the mother to her son – is an enormous factor contributing to development.

There is currently growing interest in, and much debate about, theoretical developments within the person-centred world and its application. Discussions on the theme of Rogers' therapeutic conditions presented by various key members of the person-centred community have recently been published (Bozarth and Wilkins, 2001; Haugh and Merry, 2001; Wyatt, 2001; Wyatt and Sanders, 2002). Mearns and Thorne have recently produced a timely publication revising and developing key aspects of person-centred theory (2000). Wilkins has produced a book that addresses most effectively many of the criticisms levelled against person-centred working (2003). It seems to me that the relational component of the person-centred approach, based on the presence of the core conditions, is emerging strongly as a counter to the sense of isolation that frequently accompanies deep psychological and emotional problems, and the increase in what I would term a 'rabid inauthenticity' within materialistic societies as we enter the 21st century.

This is obviously a very brief introduction to the approach. Person-centred theory continues to develop as practitioners and theoreticians consider its application in various fields of therapeutic work and extend our theoretical understanding of developmental and therapeutic processes. At times it feels like it has become more than just individuals; rather it feels like a group of colleagues, based around the world, working together to penetrate deeper towards a more complete theory of the human condition. It is an exciting time.

CHAPTER 1

Counselling session 1: beginnings and introductions

1 September

Michael worked privately for a couple of employee assistance programmes through which he received most of his referrals and saw most clients at a therapy centre. He also had a session at an NHS surgery locally. He enjoyed the contrasting work, a mixture of short-term and longer-term working and with a variety of issues: work-related, health-related and through his private work a quite diverse range. He had come into counselling after attending a workshop on relationship and listening skills. His interest had been sparked in the whole notion of 'therapeutic relationship' – what did it mean, how did it work? Following a general training course he had decided to focus on the theory and practice of the person- or client-centred approach. It was the one that he felt at home with. It fitted well with his own developing thoughts around the healing and transformative power of relationship, that if people are psychologically and emotionally damaged by unhealthy relational experiences then surely there was a case for healthy relational experience to offer a healing process. The therapeutic power of a relational experience with someone who was offering authenticity, warm acceptance and empathy struck a chord. It made sense. And his own experience in his training and therapy served to reinforce this idea.

He was due to see his new client, Peter, who had referred himself privately and they had met the previous week for a brief session. Peter had found Michael's name on the British Association for the Person-Centred Approach (BAPCA) website. He'd reached a point in his life where he wanted change. He knew he wasn't happy. He'd been doing some searches for counselling and the site had come up on the listing. He rather liked the information about what was being described – something called the person-centred approach. It sounded non-threatening. He didn't want someone endlessly analysing his every word, and he didn't want someone telling him what to do. He just felt he needed a bit of space to talk to someone, make sense of things, make some changes perhaps.

Peter had contacted Michael and they had agreed to have that preliminary session, so that Michael could explain what counselling was, what he could offer, how he worked, and for them to agree whether they felt they could work together. Michael had felt good about Peter from the start although he had been struck immediately by his hesitancy and seeming lack of confidence.

What had emerged was that Peter was struggling in many areas of his life: work, relationships, family matters. Peter hadn't given all the details but Michael was left feeling that there were unspoken concerns and he was left speculating as to what they might be. He didn't make any comment at the time; he trusted his clients to introduce topics, experiences, concerns when they felt ready and able to do so. He didn't push his clients along and certainly was not into directing them towards something that was simply speculation on his part. He strongly believed in the therapeutic potency of the non-directive element within the person-centred approach. So as he now waited for Peter to arrive for their first counselling session he was aware that his thoughts had drifted back to that previous meeting.

An essential feature of the person-centred approach to counselling and therapy is its non-directive nature. Indeed Carl Rogers, who formulated this theoretical approach, initially placed emphasis on the non-directive element. Merry (2002) cites Rogers' book, *Counselling and Psychotherapy: newer concepts in practice* (1942), as the publication in which 'Rogers' own emphasis and "non-directive counselling" became visible'. Rogers (1942) made the point that 'nondirective counselling is based on the assumption that the client has the right to select his own life goals, even though these may be at variance with the goals that the counsellor might choose for him' and that 'the nondirective viewpoint places a high value on the right of every individual to be psychologically independent and to maintain his psychological integrity'. Within person-centred therapy the client is allowed the space and time to take their own direction, to introduce the material that they wish to into the session and, at their own pace, to draw their own conclusions, attribute their own meanings and interpretations, within the warm, relational acceptance offered by the person-centred counsellor.

Michael had sensed that Peter had been quite guarded, not that that was particularly unusual. Clients often held back, particularly if for whatever reason they were not comfortable with trusting other people. After all, why should he, a perfect stranger. He felt he would need to earn Peter's trust. So, he sat and waited, glancing at the clock and noting that the time for the start of the session had nearly arrived.

The intercom buzzed; it was the receptionist.

'Your client has arrived, Michael.'

'Thanks. I'll come out to him.'

Michael walked out of the counselling room and down the corridor to the reception area. Peter was sitting, somewhat awkwardly perched on the edge of the seat.

He was dressed in rather a mixture of unmatching colours and altogether seemed somehow incongruous in some way. He stood up immediately he saw Michael. 'Er, hallo.'

'Hi, Peter, come on through.' Michael nodded an appreciation to the receptionist as he followed Peter along the corridor. 'First room on the right, like last week.'

Where there is a walk to the counselling room, who goes first? Often the counsellor will lead the way, yet sometimes the client may be invited to walk in front. It may not seem significant, but it can be. It is always worth the counsellor checking what the client prefers.

Peter entered the room and sat down in the soft blue chair on the right. He noted the small table with the lamp on it, the two pictures on the walls and the curtains that were drawn across the window, a darker blue that matched the carpet. It all seemed very ordered and somehow enhanced his own sense of disorderliness, although he wasn't thinking in quite those terms. The reality was, for Peter, that he simply felt uneasy and unsettled, unsure of what he was doing. He was nervous, well, anxious was perhaps more accurate. He'd come straight from work – hadn't said anything at home about where he was going, just that he was working late. Knew he'd get an interrogation if he'd said anything. Just felt he needed to get some space for himself, think things through, make sense of himself.

Michael had sat down opposite him. He heard him comment on what he had said the previous week about confidentiality and that he hoped Peter would find it helpful to use the time they had, and that it was his time to bring whatever he wanted to the counselling sessions.

Peter could feel his heart thumping a little more, and he felt a kind of cold sweat breaking out. He'd felt that way the previous week, though somehow this was worse. He'd met Michael and they had talked generally about counselling, what he could offer, all the practical details really. Now, well, now it was for real. Now he had to try and use this time, but in truth he didn't know how. He didn't know what to say or how to say it. He just knew he felt his life was miserable, going nowhere and he knew he needed to make some change, but felt unable to do so.

Peter was aware of the silence that had followed Michael's voice and his last comment: 'So, how can I help?'

Peter sat; he was looking at the picture on the wall opposite – a vase of yellow flowers. He could feel himself counting the petals on one of the flower heads. He brought his attention back though he wasn't sure what to focus on.

'I – er, well, I'm not sure what to say or where to begin.'

He watched Michael nodding in response. 'Mhmm, hard to know where to start, what to say – kind of difficult to begin.' He spoke fairly quietly though clearly, and waited. He could see Peter's discomfort – at least, that was how he interpreted his facial expression and body language. He thought about responding to the non-verbal communication but set it aside, at least for the moment. He didn't want to direct Peter into his body language when, perhaps, a thought process or a feeling might be emerging that was different. So he waited, taking a deep breath as he did so.

Peter heard Michael breathing deeply. He sighed. 'Where to begin? Guess it's a long story. You've no doubt heard it many times from other people ...'

'I've heard many stories but yours will be unique to you. I'd really like to hear whatever you feel you want to say.' Michael meant what he said. It wasn't, for him, some standardised counselling response. He didn't believe in that.

A key factor in person-centred counselling is that the counsellor speaks from their own genuineness within the therapeutic relationship. What Michael says here may be the same words as another therapist might use, but what is important is that they are meant, they are congruent. Michael recognises Peter's uniqueness, it is real to him, and he genuinely wants to hear what Peter has to say.

Peter sensed a genuineness in Michael's voice, almost as though he really did want to hear. But no, that was stupid, no one was really that interested, not in him. And yet ...

Michael waited. He knew how sensitive these open moments of a counselling session could be, how tempting it could be to push the client into talking, or to give them a focus by unwittingly directing them in some way – which could simply be motivated from an unrecognised desire in the counsellor to reduce tension. The need for the counsellor to know him or herself, to be able to discern what is present and why, while remaining responsive to the client, he knew could be challenging. But that was part of the professional discipline of applying the person-centred approach to therapy.

'I'm 28, still living at home and feeling, I don't know, like I just don't have a life I can call my own.' The words kind of blurted out when they came, leaving Michael very affected by the intensity of what was being said. Michael nodded, but did not have a chance to say anything. Peter was continuing. 'It's like, I don't know ...' He returned to silence and stared at the curtain. Peter had protruded his lower lip as he sat there, his mouth closed. There was tension in his upper lip as he clamped it down. He took a deep breath. He was feeling cold inside, like a damp mist had descended inside the pit of his stomach.

'Sounds painful, not feeling you have a life of your own.' Michael noted the seeming tension in Peter's facial expression. He felt that edge in himself that he often felt with a new client who was starting out to share his life and his concerns. Never being quite sure how the counselling relationship would develop and what material would emerge left Michael with that sense of raised tension inside himself that was familiar. He didn't feel a need to try and lose it; in a way it told him that, for him, he was focused and connecting with his client.

Peter heard the words but he was in another place. His mind had drifted back to an incident earlier in the week. He'd gone out with a woman from work – Melanie – they'd gone to the pictures for the evening. It wasn't something Peter often did, but, well, he'd decided he needed to do something. It had sort of followed on from booking himself in for the counselling sessions. That had somehow made him feel a little different, like he was taking some kind of control, or something, back in his life. Like he was doing something for himself. So he'd asked her out and they'd gone out after work. He'd said he'd be late back. In fact he was later than he had expected – they'd gone for a meal before the film. Ended up watching a later showing. He'd really enjoyed himself, and it had been a good film too. And then he'd dropped Melanie back home – she shared a house with some other female friends – and then headed off home himself.

The moment he'd walked through the door he'd got grief. 'So, where have you been? What time do you call this? I've been worrying about you. You said you'd be back before now.'

Peter could feel the pleasure of his evening melt away, like it just dissolved into the ether and from feeling good and having a warm smile, he suddenly felt so small, and so desperately unhappy. It was not a new feeling and one that he experienced all too frequently. And yet, in the context of his evening, this time it seemed more acute.

He'd tried to explain but his mother didn't want to know, didn't want to acknowledge that he, Peter, had enjoyed his evening. It was all about her, what effect it had had on her. Even though he had said he'd be late, clearly being later than expected was unacceptable. He went to his room and wondered why on earth he was still in the same house as her. He knew he didn't need to be. He had a good job, he could afford to move out, move on, but he never had. Suppose it had all become something of a habit, though he had been flicking through the property pages, and was considering at least renting something for himself, something small, somewhere he could call his own.

'You look so lost in your thoughts, Peter.' He heard Michael's voice. It brought him back into the counselling room.

'Oh, yes, sorry, miles away.' He smiled weakly. It somehow seemed hard to tell Michael about his thoughts. He wasn't sure why. Maybe because he was a man. But then, well, he wasn't too sure that he could have told a woman either.

'Is it something you'd like to talk about?' Michael made the invitation. He knew that he was perhaps encouraging Peter to maybe feel obliged to talk about his thoughts, and yet he justified it in that he wasn't taking Peter's focus away from what he was experiencing, merely inviting him to bring it visibly into their relationship in the room.

'Oh, it's my mother, that's what it's all about. She just can't stop interfering in my life, telling me what to do, what not to do. Always organising me, telling me what I like, what's good for me. And she can be so critical – particularly when we are alone. When other people are there, she seems to be constantly singing my praises, though usually with reference to herself, how she has helped me be successful in my work, how she brought me up to not have the kind of problems that others have.' He shook his head. 'Wish I had a few problems – life might be a bit more bloody exciting.' He looked up. 'Sorry.'

'It's OK, you'd like your life to be a bit more bloody exciting.' Michael matched Peter in his tone of voice, a kind of frustrated yearning for something, anything, to be different.

Matching tone of voice is an important element in empathic responding, along with matching the actual use of language, particularly where words are spoken with intensity. A client swears; does the therapist use the same language? What if it is language the counsellor finds offensive? Where possible, keep with the client's language. If the counsellor cannot, then for reasons of congruence this may need to be highlighted to the client and/or taken to supervision. It must not be forgotten that the client chooses the words they need to use to describe their inner world. The therapist needs the client to know that they have been heard. However, where the content of what is being said is genuinely offensive to the counsellor – racist or sexist comments, for instance – then the counsellor is at liberty to acknowledge the client's view but may well want to express their own, particularly if what is being said is impacting on the counsellor's ability to listen to the client and to experience warmth towards them.

Peter nodded. 'Yes. I mean, my life, what is it? I go to work. Yes, I'm good at what I do. Computer programmer for a biggish company. Complex stuff, you know? Good money. I enjoy it. Come home, eat, watch TV, maybe read a book, or perhaps work on something – I build electronic equipment at home, always been interested in it. I go out a little, but not often. May sometimes meet up with a couple of friends, well, maybe more acquaintances, who are in the same business but for other companies – we were at school together and are still in the same area, funnily enough. But we're not really close. They're both married now, one's got children. Me, I don't know, never really moved on somehow. Feel stuck. Sort of in a rut, I guess.'

'Mhmm, feels like a rut, huh?' Michael did not bother with a lengthy empathic reflection of what Peter had said. He preferred to stay with where the client was when he paused. Peter was engaging with the notion of being in a rut in the moment so that was what Michael responded to.

Peter nodded. 'Yes, feels like I've been there for too long as well, I guess.' He smiled wryly. 'Yeah, guess I didn't get away quick enough.'

Michael was aware of an instinctive frown on his face, a natural reaction to his wondering what Peter meant. He felt he needed to explain. 'Guess I'm curious as to what you mean by that.'

Peter had noted Michael's response and had already taken it as an invitation to explain himself, before Michael had spoken. 'Well, my brother, Barry, he left home, well, as soon as he was able really. Joined the army and got away. My sister, Lucy, followed a couple of years later – she met up with someone, they lived together for a while – mother didn't approve – kept interfering.

Anyway, they're in Australia now. And that leaves me, like I say, didn't get away. I suppose it was my father dying, I mean, I was 19 at the time. I'd left school and was starting work with an electronics company. He died – car accident. Well, I guess I felt I needed to be around for my mother. It was a hell of a shock for her, well, for all of us really, although he'd always been quiet somehow, in the family, you know? That was how he was. My mother sure wore the trousers in our house. So, like I say, I got stuck.' He took a deep breath and sighed. 'And I still am.'

There was something sad about the way Peter looked as he was speaking, He was looking down, his head slightly bowed, his hands palm down on his thighs. He looked somehow pitiful, the word that came to Michael's mind was 'pathetic' – not in any way a judgement, but somehow the word just felt like it was present in the room.

'Left at home, unable to break free to create a life of your own.'

'Pathetic, isn't it?'

Michael was glad he hadn't voiced what he had experienced, pleased to hear Peter voice the feeling.

'That's how it seems to you, Peter, pathetic.'

'Well, it is, isn't it? I mean, here I am, a grown man, and yet I can't really move on and leave her. I mean, what would her life be like then?'

'Mhmm, that's what stops you, wondering what her life would be like.'

'She's not that old, well, not old at all, and yet somehow she seems old.' He could see her as a very lonely woman if he left. She did go out – she had friends – well, he was never sure if they were real friends, but she met up with them from time to time. She had a part-time job in a small local shop, though it seemed to him that it was her way of keeping in touch with the local gossip. She had a pension from her husband's company and there had been an insurance payout as a result of the car accident, so she wasn't in any financial difficulty, and could easily live off her income and the interest if he did leave.

'She seems old?'

'Hmm? Sorry, another train of thought.'

'Maybe the other train of thought is more important to you?'

Peter took a deep breath. 'I don't know. Thinking about how it would be if I left, moved on. I know I can do it, but, well, she is my mum and I do wonder how she would react.'

'Mhmm, yes, just how would she react if you left?' Michael tried to voice his empathic response as a statement but it still came out with a kind of questioning tone.

'I don't think she'd let me get away that easily, you know?'

Michael nodded. 'It would be difficult then, for you?'

'Some days I can see it happening, other days I just somehow make excuses and, well, I guess she never really got over my father dying the way that he did. She still goes to the grave regularly. Never talks much about it. Wish she would, probably do her good, come to someone like you.'

Michael was nodding slightly. 'Quite a shock for her to recover from and it sounds like she's never really let something go, never talked.'

'Yes. But then, well, maybe I haven't either. Not that I was . . .' He thought about it. He was going to say that he wasn't that close to his father, but a memory had surfaced. It was his father who had got him into electronics, had bought him a 'build your own radio' kit when he had been about 10 or 11. Too young to really understand and yet he'd been fascinated by how, when you linked up all these components, you could tune in and pick up music. It had just captivated him somehow. His father had been one for electronics as well – but somehow, although he'd always been encouraging, he'd never felt that close to his father. It always seemed that his father escaped into his hobby, and he preferred to be on his own. But from time to time they'd spend time together. He'd go to his father for help with something and he always seemed to have the answer. But he had somehow never *felt* close; that was how it had been.

'Not that you were . . . ?'

'I was going to say "not that we were that close", but somehow maybe we were, but never really got to express it much. Never felt that close to him.' Peter took a deep breath. 'I'm not sure things would really be that different if he were still around although I guess I would have left home by now. But if I hadn't, well, I guess he'd have been the same, still somewhat remote in many ways, still dominated by my mother.'

The session continued with Peter describing more of his life at home, talking about his brother and sister, and the lives that they had now. He realised he was envious of them. Talking about them brought this out and yet he also sensed that it felt wrong to have those feelings. They'd made their decisions, he'd made his – and he knew that somehow he couldn't really leave his mother – not really, not go to the other side of the world, anyway, like Lucy had. Barry was in Wales now, firmly established with a life and family of his own.

The session ended with Michael checking out whether the session had been useful and whether it was the kind of process that Peter had wanted or expected. Peter said that it had left him still confused with many mixed feelings, but that he was determined to persevere. He felt he needed to unload, talk things through, make sense of himself and maybe gain some strength to make different choices in his life. Yet as he voiced this he could also feel himself shrinking back. 'It feels important for me to be here even though I have no idea where it will lead me. But I have to start talking, and I have to start changing.'

'Maybe that process has begun, Peter, small steps, starting to talk. Not easy.'

The agreement was to meet up weekly. Peter could feel a sense of lightness as he left the counselling session. He knew he'd get hassle when he got home, but he was determined to preserve what he felt as he drove through the darkened streets. He didn't know what made him think it, but he sensed that a journey had begun. Yes, he didn't know where it was going to lead, but somehow it felt like he had to take it. It wasn't a choice, not really. Something, somehow, demanded that he start this process and that now was the right time. Yes, he thought, there is a rightness to this, whatever may be said to me. He'd reached his street, turned and indicated to drive across the road into the driveway. The hall light was on as he entered. He could feel his anxiety rising once more. He felt his jaw tighten as he resigned himself to his fate.

Counselling session 2: 'Seen and not heard'

8 September

Peter had already started talking about his week, how he had been affected by the last session, and the contrast in his feelings between when he had left the session, and when he had got back home.

'Didn't tell her where I'd been, but she suspected I wasn't at work. I could see it in her face. Made me feel uncomfortable. You know how atmospheres can change? Well, she really didn't seem to be too pleased.' He sighed heavily.

'It really does get to you, doesn't it?' Michael sought to empathise with the sigh and hold him in his reaction.

Peter was tight-lipped. He shook his head. 'She's OK really.'

Michael hadn't expected such a sudden switch to occur and he was aware of feeling momentarily taken aback. 'She's OK?'

'Well, you know, she's had to cope with a lot and, well, you know, I mean she can be a real pain, but she does care.'

'Mhmm. She's a pain but you feel that she really cares.'

Peter did feel that, well, not so much felt it as kind of hoped for it really. The truth was, and he hadn't really appreciated this, that he had for some while found ways of making himself believe that she cared even though clearly she didn't. Small appreciative comments and actions from her he made out to be large. But the bigger, negative stuff, he tried to minimise. His sense of her caring was more in his head than a feeling. It was the product of how he interpreted her behaviour. He'd convinced himself over the years that she cared and now, well, now it was part of him. 'Yes, she cares, she looks after me, I know she has my best interests at heart.'

Michael nodded; he sounded genuine in what he was saying, and yet it didn't seem to have a ring of truth about it. Michael responded to what Peter had said. 'So you have a real sense of her having your best interests at heart?'

Peter nodded. Yes, he thought, she does. He couldn't really bring himself to criticise her. Yes, she'd given him grief during the week, but he knew she was OK really. It was how she was. But as he sat and thought about it he could feel a creeping unease deep inside of himself. He didn't like it and switched his thinking.

Is Peter accurately interpreting his inner world at this point? Or is he screening off feelings that are uncomfortable, nagging doubts as to whether his mother does really care? Peter is incongruent. He is not experiencing himself fully or accurately. Difficult feelings and thoughts are present within himself – but he is choosing not to engage with them or allow them to affect his perception of his mother. These are likely to be familiar feelings going way back into his past, and which he has developed an habitual pattern of disregarding. Yet they are there and will continue to provide seeds of discomfort until they are recognised and dealt with.

'I've got to get on with my life, get out more, I guess, I'm sure she'll understand. Just need to explain to her that I need more from my life.' As he spoke he was aware that he hadn't convinced himself but he wanted to remain positive. He could feel that unease was coming back at him again. It had become more present over recent months, and was one of the factors that had pushed him towards his decision to come to counselling.

'Yes, you feel sure she'll understand when you tell her.' Michael realised that he hadn't really empathised, but directed Peter more towards his expectation of telling her. He didn't give it any more thought. Peter's expressed need to get on with his life was not responded to.

Peter was quiet, he wanted to be positive, and yet he knew he had his doubts. He'd gone away in the past for a few days at different times, and it had never been easy. She'd make sure she called him on his mobile and there was an expectation that he would call her each day, which he did. In one sense he hadn't thought much about it, just did it, but he had become increasingly irritated by it as well.

'She's pretty strong, doesn't take "no" very easily.'

'Your mum, strong and doesn't accept "no"?'

Peter nodded. 'She just doesn't really listen, not when it's against what she wants or thinks, or believes. Just seems to always get things her way. It just happens like that.'

Michael could feel the temptation to ask for an example but held back, seeing this as not being very non-directive. Peter would tell him if he wanted to. He kept his response brief and focused on what had just been said. 'Mhmm, that's how it happens, feels like she always gets her own way, doesn't listen.'

'It's not so much that, though, it's that she always has to be right.'

'She's always right . . .'

'. . . and I'm always wrong. Well, maybe not always, but I don't get much praise.'

Michael was struck by what Peter had said. He felt sad at the thought of Peter not feeling he got praise. It was a genuine human response within himself. Yes, he was touched. It seemed an important statement somehow, as though in that moment something really important had been said. 'You don't get much praise, that seems really important and I genuinely feel saddened by that.' Michael was being transparent, he wanted to communicate his sudden experience of sadness and he knew that his own imagination was telling him that perhaps Peter had never had much praise in his life.

Peter could feel himself going quiet and his own discomfort was increasing. He did feel sad but he also didn't feel he wanted to show it. He wasn't sure what would happen, how Michael would react. He didn't like the idea of getting emotional in front of another man. Didn't feel right, somehow. Not what you did. His thoughts had gone back to his father. He'd never shown any signs of emotion, just got on with his life. Retreated to his workshop when things were difficult.

Michael was aware that Peter had gone quiet again, and he simply waited, maintaining contact with his own feelings about what had been said. Not getting much praise and feelings of sadness. A powerful experience. Michael felt a sense of compassion for Peter in his struggle. Sons and mothers, he thought to himself, a relationship that could be so beautiful for some people, but for others an absolute nightmare. Exactly where Peter's experience fitted on that continuum he wasn't sure, but he could feel in himself a sense that it was probably tending towards the nightmare end. He realised he had drifted into his own thoughts momentarily and brought his focus back to Peter who was sitting looking down, as he had done before, hands palm down on his thighs.

Michael felt a sudden urge to offer some praise to Peter. It arose from somewhere deep within himself and he had learned to trust these impulses when they emerged at times when he felt he was in close connection with a client. However, he was unsure, he had drifted away from Peter. Was this urge something of his own need to feel good about offering praise, a kind of rescue attempt to help Peter feel good about something? Or was it something else, one of those more mysterious urges to speak or act that he remembered Carl Rogers writing about, which he suggested emerged when there was a deep, inner connection within the therapist?

> 'When I am at my best, as a group facilitator or as a therapist, I discover another characteristic. I find that when I am closest to my inner, intuitive self, when I am somehow in touch with the unknown in me, when perhaps I am in a slightly altered state of consciousness, then whatever I do seems to be full of healing. Then, simply my *presence* is releasing and helpful to the other. There is nothing I can do to force this experience, but when I can relax and be close to the transcendent core of me, then I may behave in strange and impulsive ways in the relationship, ways which I cannot justify rationally, which have nothing to do with my thought processes. But these strange behaviours turn out to be *right*, in some odd way: it seems that my inner spirit has reached out and touched the inner spirit of the other. Our relationship transcends itself and becomes a part of something larger. Profound growth and healing and energy are present.' (Rogers, 1980, p. 129)

Michael was aware of a strong sense of compassion towards Peter; though his thoughts had drifted, his feelings were very present. He knew he couldn't really apply normal logic to the situation; he either had to trust the urge or let it pass, to be not acted upon. He decided to speak, his heart had begun to thump and this was often a sign to him that what he was contemplating saying was important to express.

'Well I think you're courageous coming to counselling; it isn't easy to face up to and talk about difficult experiences, choices, decisions. I want you to know that's how I feel.'

Peter had raised his eyes and was looking intently at Michael. They sat, maintaining the eye contact for some while. Michael could feel his heart still thumping. It felt an important moment but he wasn't really thinking about it or anything else for that matter. He was simply holding himself – or was he being held – in the moment.

Peter was experiencing a strange reaction. He wasn't at all sure what he felt. It sort of felt good and yet somehow didn't feel right, and yet it felt so important to have heard what Michael had said. Then again, he could also feel himself questioning the validity of what he had said. So many reactions. He also felt quite emotional as well, aware that he had a lump in his throat, which had also gone dry. Michael had felt really genuine in what he had said. It had taken Peter by surprise. He wasn't used to someone saying something like that about him, and to him, to his face, in such a direct way. The truth was that he didn't know what to feel or know how to respond. It felt good, but it felt weird. He opened his mouth but didn't know what to say. He closed it again.

Michael responded, a little speculatively, 'A lot of feelings maybe but hard to put them into words.'

Yes, thought Peter, that summed it up. He guessed that Michael had been here with many other clients. He was stepping away – without realising it – from accepting that what Michael had said was personal and specific to him. Silence reigned as both men sat facing each other. Peter, however, could feel that creeping uneasiness within himself getting stronger. He felt his body going kind of cold, like a cold sweat. He felt things and yet felt numb at the same time. Like he was feeling and not-feeling at the same time. He wasn't sitting rationalising it in this way, he just knew he felt odd, spaced out, sort of strangely present and yet detached within himself – light and heavy at the same time. He couldn't bring himself to speak; in truth he wasn't trying. He didn't feel he had anything to say. He sat passively and yet somehow, somewhere deep inside himself he was anything but passive, but it was safely distant.

Michael was sensing unease. He was experiencing its presence but he couldn't really distinguish where it was coming from. Was it something about the silence that was provoking it in him, or what had been talked about? He didn't want to speculate and thereby take his attention away from Peter yet he wanted to keep closely in touch with his own experiencing. He had encountered these moments before. They always somehow seemed particularly challenging to him, particularly as a person-centred therapist. He stayed with the sensations that had become present for him. It wasn't a discomfort, but a kind of sense that all was not well. Peter was sitting apparently quite calmly, not moving, looking down slightly, hands neatly in his lap. He found himself wondering how familiar this pose was. The thought struck him that it was the kind of pose that in another era you might have struck when visiting a great-aunt, when you had to be seen but not heard. Was that what Peter had experienced? He found the image lodging in his mind; it was hard to push it away. He thought back to his own childhood momentarily and, yes, he could relate to it. So maybe it was his stuff. He'd sat like that when he'd visited his aunt Dora. Sitting on the chair in the corner. Couldn't even swing his legs.

Michael brought his train of thought to an end and refocused back on Peter, though making a mental note to explore this in supervision. Nevertheless, the image stayed with him – the 'be seen and not heard'. Another thought came to mind, which he sensed was pushing a smile to his lips. Yes, he thought, and Peter is very much sitting here in front of me, visible and silent, seen and not heard. He felt his heart thump as the thought had struck him. Again an irresistible urge to express his thoughts. He didn't deliberate but decided to trust the urge.

'I'm not sure what you're experiencing, Peter, and I'm curious, but I do know I have a strong sense of a small boy being seen and not heard, and maybe that has no relevance but it is very present for me.'

Peter closed his eyes. As Michael spoke he was suddenly flooded with memories, and he could feel the goosebumps breaking out on his neck and up his scalp, spreading as well across his shoulders. Sitting at that damned tea-table, he could see the table-cloth and those place mats – horrible pink flowers. Having to all sit there silently – and they all had, everyone. Well, he had, and so had Lucy, but he remembered Barry rebelling. His mother gave him hell but something in him just wouldn't accept it. They would sit and listen and watch, saying nothing. He guessed it had all contributed to Barry getting away as soon as he could. The images were vivid and the feelings ... Peter let out a deep breath; he hadn't realised he had been holding it in. He took a deep breath. The unease had kind of become focused in his solar plexus and his face felt suddenly very cool. In fact he felt quite faint. He wanted a glass of water. But he couldn't ask for it. He wanted to ask for it. But something was stopping him. It was crazy, why not ask for it, but no, he couldn't. He suddenly felt very faint. He swallowed and sat back in the chair, raising his head up as he took another deep breath.

Michael had seen the colour drain from Peter's face. 'You look like you could do with a glass of water.'

Peter nodded.

Michael went out to get one for him, and handed it to him on his return. Peter took it gratefully and sipped at it, then gulped it down. He took another deep breath then had to suppress a burp. He closed his eyes and blinked a few times. He could feel the faintness lifting.

'You OK? You lost a lot of colour just then.'

'Felt faint suddenly.' Peter nodded his head slowly and almost imperceptibly. 'When you said about the little boy not being heard – yes, that was it, that was me. Ooh, I can feel the goosebumps again as I say it. That really has got to me.' He was taking another deep breath. Now he was shaking his head. Another deep breath which he blew out and promptly yawned.

'The little boy not being heard, that's what set off the goosebumps, yes?'

Peter nodded, still taking deep breaths. 'Had a lot of that. That was how it was at home. That was how it was ...' Peter's voice trailed off and to Michael it seemed like he had gone back into his thoughts, into his memory or perhaps a specific memory from his past. He empathised with what Peter had said, keeping the focus and speaking softly so as not to disturb what Peter was experiencing.

'... how it was.' Michael was aware that he had tightened his lips. He momentarily thought about how that physiological reaction was itself an expression of blocking speech. He waited for Peter to continue if he wanted.

Peter sort of snorted. 'Not how it was, sometimes feels like it never ended.'

'Like it's still that way?'

'Sometimes.' Peter paused. 'She just has to have her own way, has to keep telling me what I want, what I like, how it should be. And, you, I go with it. I feel like I've been trained to accept it, and it feels comfortable and yet I hate it too. I mean, she cooks the same things, and often on the same nights, you know? You can tell the day by what's on the plate. And, yes, part of me likes that – guess I'm so used to it – but I hate it too, hate it. Hate that bloody dinner-set, those knives and forks we've had for years. At least the bloody table-cloth's changed . . .'

Michael noted that Peter's language had become a little more colourful and passionate.

'. . . and those place mats have long since worn out.' The tone changed. 'But she means well, she's got my best interests at heart.' He looked at Michael and smiled. 'She means well, I shouldn't be critical. It's her way. She's OK really.'

Michael again noted the sudden switch. He's really split, Michael thought, switching fast from what sounded like a lot of angst to acceptance of how it was and is.

'Mhmm, in spite of what you have been saying about "telling the day by what's on the plate" and that "bloody dinner-set", you also say "she means well" and has your best interests at heart.' He felt tempted to comment that it was quite a range of reactions, but knew he would be directing Peter towards the range rather than leaving him free to focus on whatever aspect of that range of feeling was present for him, or perhaps something else may have emerged into his experience.

The non-directive element to person-centred therapy is subtly applied. Michael is struck by the range but he does not need to tell Peter this. There might also be a temptation to comment on the contrasts in what has been said, but again, that is the counsellor's experience, not necessarily the client who may, in saying what he has said, have some other more significant meaning that he might wish to explore.

Peter nodded, tight-lipped himself now. 'Yes.' He lapsed into silence, unsure what to say next. Yes, it was how Michael had said it, well, how he himself had said it too. 'She's become so stuck in her ways. It's my father dying – she hasn't got over it. Seems like she just lives her routine, she's stuck, in a rut, and I'm stuck there too. I want to get out, but I can't.'

'You can't get out of the rut?'

Peter shook his head. 'I can't.' He closed his eyes and rubbed his forehead, drawing his hand down his face. He looked over his hand to Michael. Again he felt his lips tighten.

Michael momentarily wondered whether to respond in the first or second person – he went for the second person, although he knew that it often seemed more direct and powerful for the client to hear what they had asserted. However, sometimes responding in the second person could be experienced as someone telling them how it was and this could release some other response, or a defence, or encourage a fuller experience of what had been asserted. 'You can't.' Michael waited, seeking to remain open to Peter, to what was present in the relationship that was building between them, and to himself.

For Peter it simply left him more in touch with that part of himself that was used to reacting to 'don't do that', 'you can't do that', or 'you mustn't do that': phrases he had heard many times over the years, though particularly in childhood. Now it tended to be more 'you don't want to do that', or 'you wouldn't like that', or 'that's not the way to do it'. He was taking another deep breath and sighing again.

Michael felt the struggle that was present for Peter. He sought to communicate his empathy of what had been said, sensing that the focus had not moved although in fact it had. 'You can't get out of the rut.'

'I want to say "no, I can't", but I want to as well.' He was looking into Michael's eyes now. Michael witnessed such a powerful wave of feeling in that moment – despair, sadness, a look of pleading for help.

'Yeah, want to say "no", and so desperately wanting to say "yes".'

Peter nodded.

Michael had noted a little while back that time was passing, and, yes, perhaps time was running out for Peter in his dilemma.

'I need to find a way of saying "yes". I have to get out of it, I have to.'

Michael nodded. It felt like Peter had connected with a strong recognition within himself of what he needed to do. Yes, a part of him was fighting against being in the rut. But another part had developed to comply with his mother's wishes, and that was strong and dominant. The battle was perhaps starting. Both aspects to Peter were valid parts within his structure of self. Both needed to be heard. Both wanted to survive.

'Mhmm, find a way of saying "yes" to getting out of it.'

Peter had glanced at the clock and noticed that his time was up.

'Feels like the place to end.' The session ended and Peter left. Something was still with him. He hadn't said anything. It had seemed silly, and yet ... The glass of water. Why hadn't he asked for it? But he hadn't been able to. Something had stopped him. But he had no idea why.

Points for discussion

- Evaluate the beginning process between Michael and Peter. What were the key elements to this in your view?
- What significant role did empathy play in these two sessions?
- How are you left feeling towards the client, Peter? Contrast this with the way that Michael has been feeling.
- At times Michael has spoken from his own inner experiencing. Has this been appropriate?

- What would you find particularly challenging to your practice about the way Peter has presented himself?
- If you were Michael, what would you be taking to supervision from these two sessions?
- Write your notes for these two sessions.

CHAPTER 2

Counselling session 3: 'I'm wondering if counselling is really right for me?'

15 September

Peter had experienced something of a roller-coaster of a week. He felt as though life was suddenly becoming more difficult. He was feeling more reactive, less accepting. It wasn't making his life very easy. He felt irritable, on edge, snappy. It tended to come out at work, but he was increasingly irritated with his mother. He couldn't make sense of it all, but he somehow kept thinking back to that last counselling session. Something had changed, shifted. Something was different. He couldn't define it. It was unsettling. He felt ... he found it hard to put into words as he thought about it. There was a kind of fragility and yet that wasn't right. Brittle, perhaps? But that didn't seem to sum it up either.

He was sitting outside the centre, a few minutes before the session was due to start. He wasn't clear what he wanted or needed to talk about, and he felt concerned that it would simply unsettle him even more. And yet, while he didn't like what he was feeling, somehow he also felt strangely more alive. And that didn't make sense; it seemed he was full of contradictions. He shook his head as if to try and clear it and blinked. 'Oh well,' he said to himself, and thought that maybe he could talk it through with Michael, that maybe what he was experiencing was somehow normal.

He opened the car door, got out, glanced to check the handbrake was on and pushed the door to, clicking his remote to lock it. He turned and walked towards the gate and along the path. He was walking slowly, still thinking. So much seemed to be happening yet it all seemed to be inside his head. He'd reached the door and rang the bell.

A few minutes later he was settled into the chair in the counselling room. Michael had asked him how he wanted to use their time. Peter told him what he was experiencing and asked if it was normal. Michael had empathised with his concern and confirmed that people had many different reactions to counselling, that he didn't feel it was for him to try and interpret it, but rather allow what was happening to occur and to be with Peter as he explored it and tried to attach his own meaning, if that was what he wanted.

> The person-centred therapist will not be seeking to interpret a client's experience, but rather will want to facilitate the client in experiencing what has become present for them, and allowing them to formulate their own understanding. It has to be noted, though, that this is a *process* and that no conclusion is likely to be final. As the client grows or changes within the therapeutic relationship, they will also be shifting in their relationship to, and perception of, what has become present in their awareness. So even the client's interpretation has to be viewed as contextual.

'I was thinking about it before I came in. And now, sitting here, there is something about feeling ...' Peter paused again. As he had started speaking he kind of thought he knew what he was going to say, but he'd lost it. It was like something that was sitting on the edge of his awareness but he couldn't grasp it. 'I can't get hold of it.' Peter was shaking his head.

'A feeling that somehow can't quite be felt?' Michael was responding to his sense of what Peter was communicating rather than the substance of his words.

Peter sat quietly with his eyes closed. He could feel that unsettling unease becoming present somewhere in the pit of his stomach. He was staring at the picture on the wall, seeing it but not seeing it. Thinking but not thinking. He could feel a sensation in his shoulders and upper arms, a kind of slight tingling, a sort of nervy feeling. He flexed his shoulder muscles and that helped to clear it. He took a deep breath.

He suddenly found himself thinking back to the last session. He hadn't planned to, but it was there, present for him, and his thoughts afterwards. The glass of water. He was aware that his throat was dry. 'Can I have some water?'

'Sure.' Michael had made sure there was a jug and two glasses in the counselling room. He reached over and poured two glasses.

'Thanks.' Peter appreciated the cool fluid passing over his tongue and down his throat. 'I wanted water last week but didn't ask for it.'

'Mhmm. That sort of stands out for you?'

Peter was nodding and looking puzzled. 'I don't really understand why. Seemed such a natural thing to do, but last week I couldn't. I felt blocked. Daft, really.'

'Mhmm, wanted to ask for water but couldn't, and there was a sense of feeling blocked in some way?'

'Can't remember exactly how it was, but I was somehow left thinking about it after the session. And I don't know why.'

Michael nodded in response. 'Don't know why.'

Peter tightened his lips. The unease was back – had it gone? He'd lost awareness of it for a bit but now it was present. He didn't like it and didn't want to focus on it. 'Guess it was nothing. One of those things. Maybe I'm feeling more relaxed here.' The tension had grown a bit more inside himself.

'Can happen, can take a while to feel at ease.'

Michael was aware of feeling that they were having a conversation around something. It didn't feel direct in some way, but he didn't want to interrupt the
process, so he stayed with Peter, waiting for him to respond.

'I'm not sure that counselling is helping. I mean, I don't seem to be making any
progress and I'm finding myself more reactive. Wasn't a good week last week.
I'm wondering if counselling is really right for me.'

Michael heard what Peter had said and sensed a certain hesitancy in his voice.
It was like what he was saying wasn't strong, wasn't wholly himself speaking.
Or was he just making an assumption, an interpretation, to fit his own thoughts
about the constitution of the person? For some while, and very much in line
with certain perspectives on person-centred theory, he regarded the structure
of self to be formed of often distinctive parts or 'configurations' as they have
been described.

Mearns (2000; Mearns and Thorne 1999) has introduced the concept of
'configurations of self'. He writes that 'a "configuration" is a hypothetical
construct denoting a coherent pattern of feelings, thoughts and preferred
behavioural responses symbolised or pre-symbolised by the person as reflective of a dimension of existence within the Self' (2000, p. 102). Patterns of
feelings, thoughts and behaviour might be thought of as clustering together
in association with a particular aspect of the person's felt existence. So, for
instance, the person who feels rejected, if this is an experience that they
have had on a number of occasions, may develop a set of reactions to this
experience. They might conceptualise it as 'rejected me' and when something happens that takes them into this particular sense of self then the
associated feelings, thoughts, behaviours are likely to emerge and be lived
out. So 'rejected me' might leave the person feeling sad, or thinking they
are worthless or behaving in a manner that provokes further rejection in
order for that part to grow and maintain its existence.

'So, part of you is really questioning being here?' Michael realised that as he was
speaking he'd introduced the idea of a part, and this was not what Peter had
conveyed, and maybe wasn't experiencing. He knew why he had done it. It had
seemed like part of Peter and he often thought of clients in terms of parts. It felt
like part of him had found a voice suddenly, for whatever reason, and perhaps
linked to the focus of the session a few minutes back – the glass of water.

'Yes, oh I don't know. I know I have to change, get on with my life, but I feel, oh I
don't know ...' Peter lapsed back into silence. 'I just,' he took a deep breath,
'I just wish I could be like other people, you know, like my brother. He's got a
life of his own now. And a family. And what do I have?' He stopped again. 'But
I can't leave her. She needs me.'

'That's how it feels, you can't go, though you want a life of your own like your
brother. Your mother needs you, you don't feel you can go.'

'It's a mess, I mean, and like I said before, at least I think I did, but maybe I didn't, I don't know. But, well, it's like I kind of accept the way it is ...' Peter had stopped again.

'Kind of accept?' Michael responded with a question as what Peter had said had sounded quite hesitant.

'Well I do.' He shrugged his shoulders. 'And some days it's fine, but more and more – and particularly since coming and seeing you – I find it hard to accept.'

'Mhmm, hard to accept being there with your mum.'

'Yes, and yet thinking about leaving, well, that's kind of scary and exciting too. I don't know – I suppose where I am, well, it's kind of cushy, you know. It's just that ...' Peter took a deep breath and sighed.

Michael empathised by taking a deep breath himself and let it out slowly in the silence. 'It's just that?'

'She irritates the hell out of me.'

Quite a significant shift. Peter is allowing himself to have ownership of his feeling of irritation. The 'part' of himself that might normally have sought to have compensated for a negative reaction has remained silent.

'Mhmm.' Michael noted to himself that this seemed to him to be the first time Peter had said something negative in relation to his mother without immediately compensating with something positive. He didn't respond immediately, allowing time for what had been said to maybe sink in. Then he empathised. 'She irritates the hell out of you.'

Peter was in his own thoughts, the sense that his life was not really his own, that he almost had to report in to her all of the time, keep her informed all the time about what he was doing. He didn't always, but it always provoked a reaction. And the put downs. How many times had he heard his mother talk glowingly about his brother, what he had achieved since he'd left home – he had his own business and was quite successful, living in North Wales. She took credit for that even though she had nothing positive to say about him when he'd been at home. Barry rarely came home, hadn't seen him for some months now.

As Peter looked back over his own life he knew that he'd always been put down in his life. It was like he was never really wanted. He felt a rush of emotion as he thought about that. Never really wanted. He'd felt that for all of his life, and yet, here he was, still with her, unable to get away. Like they were locked in some – the idea of some macabre dance, stretching towards death – he pushed the thought away.

'She doesn't really care for me, not really. She's always criticised me. I've always been the one that's "in the way". I don't understand why.'

'Sounds like it might be easier if you could understand it?' Michael was responding to the desperate tone to Peter's voice as he spoke those last four words.

Peter nodded. 'I wish I could. I'm never good enough, at least, that's what she says to me. And yet, I've heard her talk to her friends and she seems to say positive things about me, but never to my face.'

'Hmm, never good enough and yet she says something different to other people? Leaves you struggling to understand.'

Peter was nodding again. 'Exactly, that's how it is. Just can't understand why she isn't really interested in me.' He took another deep breath which he again let out slowly. 'I do feel sorry for her, genuinely, but I'm also feeling increasingly irritated and frustrated and, I don't know, I feel I can't breathe sometimes.' Peter's voice had become a little louder and it seemed to Michael that he had become a little more animated as well.

'That closed in, can't breathe.' Michael hunched up his body posture as a way to convey a kind of physical empathy to Peter's words.

> Empathy does not have to be a verbal response; a deliberate use of body posture, as in this instance, can be extremely helpful. It is highly likely that memory can be stored in association with posture, and that adopting postures can release these associated memories or emotions.

Peter responded in kind. 'Yes, like I'm sort of bowed just like that.' He assumed the posture himself. A flood of emotion hit him. It was a posture all too familiar but he hadn't thought about it in those terms until now. Standing – or sitting – shoulders hunched and looking down, feeling sorry for himself. He suddenly felt so very sad, and alone.

Michael detected a shift in the atmosphere in the room. Peter suddenly looked smaller, Michael was half expecting to hear him talk like a little boy. He'd experienced that before in therapy. It seemed that Peter was retreating into the chair, and away from him. He expressed his experience.

'It seems to leave you appearing very small.'

'I feel small . . . like I can't do anything. I-I want to run away, but I can't. I never ran away. Didn't dare. I'd wanted to. God knows I'd wanted to. Barry did, and Lucy, they ran away. I didn't. Now, well . . .' Another deep breath. The thought in Peter's head was 'and now it's too late', but he didn't say it.

'They got away, ran away, you didn't, and now . . .' Michael ended with what Peter had said, intending to hold that focus, allow Peter the opportunity to develop it if he so wished.

'And now . . .' He shook his head. He didn't know what to do now. That was the problem. And it felt like it was getting more difficult. He rubbed his right hand through his hair, rubbing his scalp. The sensation felt good. A momentary distraction, but that was all it was. He felt tired, fed up. It all seemed too much, too big. He thought about how he was at work – the contrast. He was confident there – at least, he seemed more confident. He knew what he was doing and he knew he was good at what he did. He knew it. He didn't need anyone – his mother in particular – to tell him. She never did, of course. How many times had he heard her say 'Computers!' in a tone of contempt: 'Just cause more problems. Don't know why we have to have them.'

He'd given up trying to persuade her about the value of computers long ago, but it still irritated and when he heard her saying these things – and the tone of voice was so grating on his nerves – there were times he just wanted to say 'shut the fuck up'. He never did. He guessed he probably never would. But there were times – generally afterwards – when he had those thoughts. Usually later, when he was in his room, thinking about it. It stayed as a thought.

Michael could see the intensity on Peter's face; while the minutes ticked by he sat, maintaining his empathic sensitivity as well as holding a feeling of compassion in his heart for Peter. Having this feeling present was an important element in the therapeutic process as far as he was concerned.

Having a sense of unconditional positive regard for a client contributes to the healing process. It has been described in terms of warmth, prizing, an attitude of acceptance. Empathy links the counsellor to the client, offering an opportunity for these feelings and attitudes to be held and communicated. Yet it seems that perhaps compassion goes a little beyond this, taking the counsellor's feeling for, or is it towards, their client to another depth. Compassion means entering a commonality of feeling. The client's world is entered, and that world enters into the counsellor's world. There is a necessary blurring as what is experienced by the client becomes mutual.

In some Eastern spiritual traditions distinction is drawn between the feelings of the solar plexus (the more personal, gut reaction feelings) and those of the heart (more subtle and expansive). It could be argued that the presence of compassion within the counsellor for the client and their experience is more of a genuinely heartfelt response, adding depth and offering opportunity for an emergence within the client. What form this will take will depend on many variables, but it is perhaps best described as a greater or fuller capacity to love.

Whereas empathy can be generated, and to a degree so can feelings of warmth towards a client, however, compassion is perhaps more of an emergent state that cannot be made to be present. We might say that the therapeutic process moves forward when it is present, but it cannot be made to be present by either the counsellor or the client. It emerges as a result of the quality of relationship – in terms of the core conditions – that has been generated. By offering empathy, congruence and unconditional positive regard, a climate of relationship is created within which compassion can emerge. Coupled to this, I believe, comes another emergence that is to do with a person's capacity to love and be loved.

Peter felt very much in his own thoughts – and it was in his thoughts. He spent a lot of time thinking about things, far more than feeling about them. He was aware of a sense of awkwardness now as his awareness of Michael sitting, so attentively, became more present for him. People listened to him at work when he talked about his programming. That seemed to command respect. But on any other topic, or in any other setting, he never felt listened to. Seemed weird. He didn't know what to say. He shifted in the chair.

Michael chose that moment to respond, taking the physical movement as perhaps being an outer symbol of an inner shift in whatever Peter was thinking about.

'Lot to think about, Peter?' His tone of voice invited a response.

Peter took a deep breath. 'Just thinking about you, sitting there, listening. It's unsettling.' He tightened his lips and had gritted his teeth before he relaxed a little and continued. 'Never been listened to much – except dad, sometimes. Well, that's not true. I mean, Lucy and I, well, we'd talk.' He was smiling. He could remember the times they'd talked about how it felt being at home, but then she'd got a bit older and spent more time with her friends. 'She listened. We were just kids but, well, it brought us close. Barry was already out and about with his mates.'

'So apart from your dad, Lucy was the person who listened to you?'

Peter nodded. He was reflective. 'I guess I've never talked much about feelings.' He stopped, still very much reflective and in his head. He wasn't actually too sure how to. 'I think a lot, spend a lot of time in my head. Well, work's like that too, all very logical and thoughtful.'

Michael nodded, his own mind and given him the thought that probably that was why Peter had embraced computer programming as a career – no feelings, all thoughtful.

'A lot of time in your head and somehow feelings, they don't get such a look in.'

'Not to talk about. I mean I do have feelings, you know? I'm not some kind of robot.'

'Mmm, I appreciate that.' Michael noted a slightly defensive tone in his response.

Not a very helpful response and, yes, saying more about Michael than communicating any of the content of what Peter had been saying. He could have been more empathic to Peter's affirmation of being not some kind of robot.

'Sometimes I almost wish I could feel more. It's not that I couldn't feel, but I kind of sense that other people, well, they kind of seem lighter somehow. Everything seems too serious to me.' He sighed. 'I do have feelings. I read the papers and different magazines, and think about the world, about the unnecessary suffering and death as the rich corporations exploit the poor and destroy environments. It makes me sad. I do feel for people, and I can feel so helpless as well. What kind of a world is this?' He had gritted his teeth and was shaking his head.

'Seems like the state of the world, the suffering, death, exploitation really touches you deeply. And, yes, it leaves you wondering – as it leaves me wondering – "What is this world all about?"' Michael was genuine in his response. He was aware that the conversation had moved on, but he trusted Peter's need for this shift of focus. Peter was talking about an area of his life that gave him strong feelings. He stayed with him.

Peter nodded.

Michael repeated what he had said, but in a slightly resigned tone. 'What is this world all about . . . ?'

They sat together in silence. Peter didn't often talk in this way, or about this kind of thing. In truth, he hadn't said much, but he had shared something of himself to Michael. He didn't often, well rarely ever, talk of these things at work. His colleagues were more concerned with the latest football results, new cars, fashions, tabloid scandals. He often felt quite critical of them. He wished he could make a difference, somehow, somewhere. Yet here he was, stuck at home, unable to move on. Sometimes he thought he'd explode with it, at other times it just all felt like a colossal heavy weight pressing down on him, stifling any possibility of movement. He didn't know what else to say now. Felt like Michael's question was one that just hung in the air. He didn't know what the world was about, but he knew that it seemed at times like a world gone mad. The silence continued.

'Just seems crazy out there and I guess it all feels too big. Difficult enough sorting my own life out, let alone the world. I'll leave that for others.'

Michael listened and knew that, if he were in normal conversation, his response would be different to the one that he gave. 'Hmm. It feels too big, too crazy. Difficult enough to sort your own life out, yes.'

> It can be an interesting exercise to look at a comment made by a client in a therapy session and contrast your counselling response with what it might be if you were having a general conversation with the person. This simple exercise can encourage the counsellor to become aware of whether, in certain instances and in relation to specific topics, his or her personal views or opinions are impacting on the quality of their empathy.

Peter nodded, and glanced at the clock, noting that the time was passing, just a few minutes of the session left. He didn't really want to get back into anything else. He was in a familiar place in himself now.

Michael had noticed the glance and he acknowledged it. 'Just a few minutes left.'

'Feels like we've covered many things today.'

'Yes, it feels like I've got to know you more, or rather got to know more of you.' Michael spoke very much from his experience of listening to Peter.

'I feel somehow more me sitting here now. Somehow calmer.' He took a deep breath and held it for a moment. 'Yes.' He let the air back out.

Michael nodded. 'And I'm conscious that earlier you talked about wondering if the counselling was helpful and I want to check out whether you plan to continue, or whether those doubts are leaving you thinking otherwise.'

> Counselling is not the answer to everything, and some people may find that they need to think seriously about the timing of entering into counselling or therapy. It can be demanding on the client. It is often helpful to discuss this if a client raises the issue. Perhaps the timing is not right, that they have other demands in their life that need addressing before they can give themselves psychological space to engage with the therapeutic process. For others, the

> need is present to have someone consistent to turn to, to talk to, a place of
> safety away from a demanding or threatening world. There is no question
> for them of postponing the therapeutic process. It can also be that the experi-
> ence of coming into counselling is not matching the client's expectations.
> This will need careful and sensitive handling to enable the client to make a
> truly informed choice as to what he or she wishes to do.

Peter shook his head. 'I want to keep coming. I feel that there's a lot I want to tell
you. I haven't talked much in my life, and haven't been listened to. It's strange.
But I somehow begin to sense that it's important to talk, yes, I need to talk.'
He smiled. 'And maybe more importantly, I need to feel heard, listened to,
you know?'

Michael did know what Peter meant. He'd often carried in the back of his mind:
'it's good to talk, but even better to feel heard.' 'Yes, I do appreciate what you
are saying. I'm glad I can listen to you. And I hope that maybe, as you get used
to it, as it becomes less strange and more familiar, then, well, who knows? But I
believe that it is helpful.'

'OK, So, same time next week. Thanks, Michael, I do appreciate your time. I feel
that this week I have a lot to think about.' He smiled grimly. 'Think about!
That's me.'

'Yes, it's a familiar place in yourself, a place you have developed and go to a lot.'

'It is. And while I don't want to lose that, I want more. Oh well, we'll see. It would
be good to know what will happen next. I mean, I like things to be structured,
I like to know what happens next. I like things to follow a kind of logical
pathway. This seems so different, and yet it does have a certain, I don't know,
something compelling about it. That hasn't really struck me until now. I'm curious. I feel weird but it also feels right as well. I don't know, I'm waffling.'

'That's how it feels to you, and I want to acknowledge that I hear something
important. You're used to logical, methodical things with clear pathways and
goals. This, well, we don't know. More of a mystery tour.'

Peter smiled. 'Yes. Life's a mystery. Maybe this brings me in touch with reality in
some way.' He paused. 'Oh well. Thanks. Time I was heading off.' He stood up
and a couple of minutes later was sitting back in his car. He still felt strangely
calm, and there was something else. It was a kind of sensation rather than a
feeling – he tried to identify what it was. It wasn't very familiar, and yet it felt
good. Felt good. That's what it was. He felt good. He was surprised at how surprised he felt about it. He heard himself saying out loud, 'Have I ever felt good?'
Well, yes, he had, but somehow not quite like this, at least, not for a very, very
long time. His thoughts were back to his childhood and the talks with Lucy.
She'd always talk about how she wanted to get married, live in a big house,
lots of children. He'd always sort of agreed but he'd struggled to really see
it happening ... But that had been a different kind of feeling good. He had
felt heard by Michael, it seemed that they had connected, he had connected.
It felt like there had been a shift and, yes, it kept coming back to that simple
word, 'good', yes, it felt, he felt, good.

He pulled on his seat belt and turned the ignition key. He was not aware that he did so with a little more determination than usual, that he was gripping the steering wheel in a slightly more purposeful way, that he accelerated away once the car began moving with a little more intensity than usual.

Michael, meanwhile, was back in the counselling room pondering on that last session. His next client had called to cancel so he had more time to reflect. They had ranged across a number of topics, and Peter had spent a lot of time in thought. And that was OK. Thoughts, feelings, they are part of our make-up, neither more important than the other. He smiled as he thought of how often counselling was seen as simply a 'feeling-centred' process. He knew it was more than that, how often clients could be directed away from their thoughts, as if the only arena for therapeutic action was the feelings. Yes, of course they were important, but many clients – like Peter – also dwelt a great deal in their thoughts, they were 'thinking beings' maybe more than 'feeling beings'. He wanted to form a relationship with his clients as they are, so that would mean entering their thought world to connect with them. Why should a client who perhaps finds feelings difficult or unfamiliar want to expose them to a stranger? No, let's build the relationship with Peter as he is – a thoughtful person – and then, in time, and when he feels safe, then maybe the feelings will be encountered and become more present within the therapeutic relationship.

> While the person-centred counsellor is seeking to form a relationship with the whole person of their client, the reality is that this is achieved by forming relationship with and through those parts of the clients that they are connected with or expressing themselves through. If a client is in their emotions then the counsellor's empathy towards that area of experiencing encourages the connection. If the client is thoughtful and reflective, then that is the point of contact and again the empathy ensures the establishing of connection.

Counselling session 4: reactions to Peter's father's death

22 September

Peter had felt even more unsettled the following week. There had been stable times, but at other times he just felt so on edge, but a kind of overwhelmed, heavy kind of sensation. It seemed to include both anxiety and a flattening of his mood, and curiously it felt almost as though they were occurring at the same time.

He was telling Michael how busy his week had been. 'Work's gone mad, crazy deadlines. I'm working longer hours to get things done. In one way that feels good – I'm not at home so much. But it brings with it anxieties and I feel so tired some nights, and some mornings. I don't sleep through, seem to have got stuck into this habit of waking up feeling anxious at 3.30am, seems to happen every night. I can now be sure of the time when I'm lying there before I open my eyes. It really is leaving me tired, and that means I'm more irritable.' He shook his head. 'I need my own space. And I'm really struggling with feelings. At times I feel desperately in need of something, some kind of caring, affection. Something, anything.' He was shaking his head again.

'That need for affection, for someone to care about you ...'

He'd been out with Melanie again; they seemed to get on really well. It had felt good to talk to her – she really did seem to listen and understand. Not that he'd said a great deal about how things were at home – in truth he felt rather embarrassed by it all.

Peter took a deep breath as he began to speak. 'And there's something else, and I don't know what it's about, but it's from a session a while back. I remember my hesitancy asking for a drink here, and somehow that really did stick with me. I mean, I can be quite withdrawn, not push myself forward, you know, that's me, but something about that got to me.'

'Got to you? I'm wondering what that means for you.' Michael was offering a kind of empathic question, an invitation to explore a little.

'Well, I give myself a hard time, you know, when I may want something, or feel I have something to say, but hold back. I've been like that, well, it seems all of my life. So it's nothing new. And yet, there was something weird about that moment here, even though it didn't really make such a huge impression at the time. But it's stuck with me. It's like I can't shake it off, and I don't know why.'

'Seems like it's really pre-occupying you, Peter, something about not being able to ask for a drink, something ...' Michael left his response mid-sentence, seeking to empathise with the unfinishedness of what had emerged into Peter's subjective focus.

'Something.'

'Do you want to spend time thinking about it to yourself, or try to zero in on it by kind of focusing in a little more through our dialogue?'

It can be really helpful to ask the client to give direction. The person-centred counsellor will want to avoid being directive, but that does not mean not emphasising a focus that has been made visible by the client, or making visible a choice where it is clear that there are at least two potential directions and the counsellor is uncertain which the client wishes to pursue.

Peter thought and smiled. 'Part of me would be happy just thinking about it, but I've done that all my life, thought about things afterwards, replayed experiences, thought of what I should have said or done, you know? Just adds to the frustration. That never solved anything. So I guess I need to talk about it and, well, that feels scary.'

'Feels scary?'

'Like, well, like I don't have control. I mean, if I keep it in my head, I keep in control in some way. But once I, well, reveal things to you, well, I don't know what will happen.'

'Scary not feeling you'll be in control and not knowing what may emerge, yeah?'

Peter was nodding, but he also knew within himself that he had to start facing up to some of these behaviours and reactions. He had spent a lot of his life in his head and while it was really familiar territory – that place in himself where he felt most at home – he also knew that there were areas of himself that needed exploration. Feelings were bubbling through in his life – not always comfortable ones as well. His mind had gone back to that earlier session, not asking for what he wanted.

Michael kind of sensed some sort of shift within the atmosphere. He guessed Peter might be thinking about something else, maybe what he had been talking about just now.

Peter could feel a heavy weight developing in his stomach, heavy, hard, solid. He didn't like it. He felt a little spaced out, like his head was all buzzy, and he felt a tension in his temples. Not asking for what he wanted. He spoke quietly, 'I just struggle to ask for what I want . . .'

Michael nodded and while maintaining his openness to the moment and with his attention on Peter, he was also aware that his mind was holding the fact that what had happened in that earlier session was that Peter had not been able to ask for a drink, more precisely, a drink of water. As he thought that he felt goosebumps breaking out on his left side, fleetingly. They had taken his attention from Peter; he brought it back, suppressing his urge to want to think more about what significance that might have had. He looked at Peter who was speaking again.

'. . . like my father.' He was shaking his head. 'Just like dad, never really got what he wanted. Maybe he thought like I did?' He shrugged. He didn't know. He suddenly felt an overwhelming surge of sadness for his father. One particular image came to mind, one particular day when his mother had really had a go at him about something, blaming him for – he couldn't remember what now. But it was something inconsequential, it usually was. He remembered his father had quietly got up and as he had walked past he had looked straight into his eyes, Peter could see them so clearly. His father had wonderful blue eyes, and they were so full of tears, so much sadness. He felt warm tears on his own cheeks. He could feel them trickling down his face, hot, his throat was suddenly incredibly dry, and he swallowed to try and moisten it, but it didn't make a difference. He saw that Michael had poured water into two glasses; they were there on the table when he had come in. He reached out for one, yet even that somehow seemed a struggle. Like he shouldn't do it. The tears were continuing to flow. He sipped the water, put the glass down and leaned back into the chair. The feeling in his stomach had moved; it was more of a general weight or pressure on his chest.

Michael was watching Peter closely and, seeing his tears and sensing his pain, moved fractionally closer. He didn't want to distract Peter but wanted to convey a sense of wanting to be there for him. He had appreciated the lack of caring and affection that Peter felt had been his experience in life. Michael could only imagine how many times Peter might have sought affection only to have someone retreat or, worse still, react negatively and shatter his genuine but ineffectual attempts to feel loved.

The room seemed to have become very silent and still. Nothing seemed to exist other than the two of them as they sat – Peter with the tears still flowing down his face, the weight on his chest, his throat dry and burning; Michael wanting to reach out with his heart to Peter. He sat, consciously centred in his feelings, trying not to think too much himself.

'I loved him.'

Michael watched Peter close his eyes as he spoke those words, and his face crumple as the tears flowed even more. Peter swallowed, trying to regain some kind of control, but he couldn't. He just saw his father's face; it was so vivid. He missed him; he hadn't realised how much he missed him. Why had he died like that? Why? It wasn't fair. He was such a good man. Why? Why? He took a deep breath.

'Why did he die, why? I was always told that God took you when He was ready, when He needed you. I don't know. He was a good man, Michael, he had so much to put up with in his life, but he carried on. He worked hard. He did so much around the house, never really getting much appreciation, but he never gave up. I don't know why. I don't understand. Why did he stay? People don't these days, do they? Why did he stay?'

Michael nodded slowly. 'Why did he stay – that question's really present?'

Peter suddenly looked horrified, his face had changed, he was suddenly alert, a mixture of horror and puzzlement. 'You don't suppose he stayed, he stayed because of me?'

These are powerful moments in therapy, when a client suddenly has a realisation about something. The person-centred counsellor will want to empathise not only with the realisation but the effect it is having on the client. They may also be affected themselves and need to deal with their own reactions. What is vital is that they convey warm acceptance of what the client is now comprehending but without directly encouraging it.

'Because of you?'

Peter was nodding slowly, his eyes suddenly wide open. 'Yes. I mean, you don't think he stayed for me, to try and be there, to kind of, well, maybe reduce the effect of my mother's critical attitude?'

'You look as though this is a new thought, could he have stayed for you, to reduce the impact of your mother's critical attitude?'

Peter was quiet. It made a lot of sense, and he was hit by another surge of emotion. His father could have left, maybe if he had left, maybe he'd still be alive.
Oh God, he thought to himself. He sacrificed himself for me. Not directly, but
somehow that had been the effect. He'd stayed ... and he'd died. Peter was
thinking back to when he'd heard his father was dead. The police had come in
the evening. His father had been working late at work and had stopped on the
way home to pick up some shopping. Peter began to tell the story to Michael.

'He'd stopped off at the supermarket after working late, January it was, the 16th.
It had been cold and frosty. He was a careful driver, but, well, he'd worked
late – maybe he shouldn't have, but he was covering someone else's shift.
Police weren't too sure what had happened, but he'd hit a lorry on the by-
pass. Could have been ice. Died instantly, they said. Why him?' Peter was shaking his head again. 'He was such a good, patient man. I can imagine him not
wanting to leave because of me, though I was 19 by then, he could have left.'
The thought struck Peter and Michael at the same time. It was Peter who
voiced it. 'He did leave.'

'Yeah, he did.' Michael kept his response simple and waited, respectful of the
moment and of the immense inner experiencing that must be taking place
within Peter. He had no wish to disturb the flow taking place within Peter's
heart and mind. They sat in silence.

Peter felt suddenly numb. He just did not know what to think or feel, or say. He just
sat, motionless, as if he was suddenly in suspended animation. He felt, well,
he didn't feel. He wasn't thinking about anything. He wasn't feeling about anything. It was like he'd entered into a psychological paralysis. Nothing moved,
nothing stirred within him. He sat. Michael sat opposite. The silence, the stillness, overwhelmed the space that they shared as they sat together.

Minutes passed. Michael noted the expression on Peter's face. The look of horror
had passed some while back. It now seemed quite blank, almost drained,
exhausted.

Peter actually felt as though someone had pulled a plug out somewhere in his
body, all his energy having gone down some energetic plug-hole. He looked at
Michael, blowing out a breath as he did so. His arms felt heavy; his neck felt
stiff. He rotated his head slightly to try and free it off.

'Quite an experience there, Peter, seems like a lot of emotions, feelings and
thoughts flooded you. You look drained.'

'Yes. Feeling really heavy. Some of the images were so clear. My dad's face, it was
so vivid, so real. I do miss him. I do think about him a lot, he had his reasons to
stay on. I'll never know what they were. He made his choices.' He paused. 'And
I've got to make mine. I can't go on living in his shadow.' He felt slightly taken
aback as he heard himself utter that last sentence.

Michael reflected it back, having also noticed the sudden change in Peter's face as
he spoke. 'Can't go on living in your father's shadow.'

'He did what he had to do.' Peter was looking down. He looked up. 'I did love him.
I do miss him. I do wonder where he is, what he is thinking, what he would want
of me now. I think he'd want me to get on and live my own life. He didn't, maybe

couldn't. I can't continue the same pattern. I have been. But it's not the way forward. I have to ...' He took a deep breath and paused, suddenly unclear what it was that he had to do. 'I have to make my own way, move on, move out. I keep saying it but somehow it feels different now. Like I know it. I mean, I knew it before, and thought I really knew it, but maybe I didn't. Something has perhaps begun to shift a bit more.' He shook his head as he thought back to the last half of the counselling session. So many feelings had flooded him, overwhelmed him, and yet, like a wave on the sea, it had passed through and moved on. It was like as it had passed through him it had carried his emotions with it. He knew that wasn't how it was, but that's what it felt like, a huge wave sweeping through him. 'I feel washed out, Michael, literally. I think I need to take time to just settle back down before heading off.'

'Seems like it was a really powerful experience for you, Peter, I don't know if it was some kind of release, but you say something feels like it has shifted, leaving you washed out.'

'And tired. And calmer.' Peter smiled. 'What is this thing called counselling? I come here, sit down, talk about things and, wham, things start happening. Is it always like this?'

It was Michael's turn to smile. 'No, not always.'

Some clients seem to arrive at counselling ready to connect with thoughts, feelings, release experiences, redefine themselves and begin a process of recreation. Often in this case, what is seeking to emerge into awareness is already beginning to press itself upon the person's consciousness; they just require the presence of a person offering the core conditions. Others are in a very different place, sometimes never fully engaging in the therapeutic process, or needing a lot of time to build the degree of trust in the therapeutic relationship that will enable them to begin to risk revealing their inner world. The person-centred counsellor is open and accepting of whatever response emerges from the client, recognising that the client must be trusted to travel at their own pace, and on their own path – sometimes it is short and direct, sometimes meandering, and oftentimes requiring the need to travel over certain sections again and again, offering opportunity for a fuller and deeper appreciation of what is being experienced.

The session drew to a close. Peter was beginning to feel a little less numbed by his experience. He was left feeling somehow more determined, more purposeful. He did feel like he had let go of something. He did feel like he was moving on, tentatively. And it did seem somehow connected to his father. He didn't understand it. His father was still very present to him as he reached his car. He spent a few minutes sitting before turning the ignition. He realised that he had determined to tell his mother about the counselling. He felt strong. He felt good. He knew it was the right thing to do and he felt that the time was right.

Points for discussion

- What were the key moments, in your view, within these last two sessions?
- Do you experience Michael as conveying unconditional positive regard for Peter, and of Peter receiving this? Can you give examples?
- What are the important elements to address with clients who are uncertain whether counselling is right for them? How would a person-centred counsellor in particular handle this?
- How would you define the right moment for someone to enter into counselling?
- If you were Peter, what would you have most valued, and found most unhelpful, in Michael's responses?
- What issues would you take to supervision from these two sessions if you were the counsellor?
- Write counselling notes for these two sessions.

CHAPTER 3

Supervision session 1

23 September

'I've a new client, a young man in his late twenties, mixture of coming to terms
with the death of his father when he was 19, and wanting to move away from
living at home with his mother.'

'You sound very matter of fact as you speak.'

'I guess I am, but there have been a lot of feelings in the sessions. Although
Peter – that's his name – talks of being in his head a lot, spending time thinking about things, the last session in particular he was really upset, really
connected with feelings towards his father who died in a car crash. Said he felt a
real shift through that experience.' Michael went on to describe Peter a little
more and his impression of him. Michael's supervisor, Suzy, was struck by a
sense that somehow Michael was holding something back as he spoke. She
couldn't quite grasp what exactly, but somehow the way Michael was speaking
seemed to have less feeling tone to the way she was used to him speaking. She
drew attention to this.

'That's interesting. You mean I'm not really conveying feelings about Peter?'

'You may be conveying them and I may not be hearing them. My sense is that
feelings are somehow not as present as they often are when you talk about
clients. I'm curious.'

Michael was frowning. He thought he had a lot of feelings about Peter. He certainly felt his sadness, and he had been very struck by a sense of his struggle
to – well, the way he, Michael, saw it – the struggle Peter had to become a
man within his relationship with his mother. So he was also a bit puzzled as
he thought he had connected to and was conveying feelings.

'I don't think you're hearing them.'

A moment's silence passed between them. 'OK, let's take some reflective time here.
What's happening? You are talking about a client, saying you feel you are in
touch with feelings, and I'm saying I can't sense them, can't respond to them.'

'That's different, you can't respond to them. That's really interesting because
that's what Peter experienced. I'm pretty sure he got very little affection as a

child – if ever. So there is every chance his feelings were not heard, at least by his mother.'

'Mhmm, and I'm not hearing them in you. How does it feel for you?'

'Irritating. Frustrating. And yet somehow there's something about not being surprised. Like this is kind of what I'd expect, the sense that feelings not getting heard is like being passed down the counselling line. I think I hear my client's feelings, but then my feelings seem to you to be lost.'

'So as you speak about Peter you feel . . . what?'

Michael opened his mouth but wasn't sure what to say. What did he feel? He knew he felt sadness for him, and anger towards his mother. Also sympathy in relation to the loss of his father. Michael had not had that experience, his father was alive, and so was his mother with whom he had a good relationship. Michael did a bit of a reality check on himself. Where was he? He thought about Peter, recalling how he was in that last session and how he, Michael, had felt. He had been left feeling quite tired although he had felt energised as well by the way Peter had engaged with his feelings. Was energised the right word? Maybe not, but it had felt good, it had felt productive and he had a real sense of connection from that session.

Michael realised he had become lost in his own thoughts, and hadn't responded to Suzy. Lost in his thoughts. He smiled. 'Maybe I'm a little too much in my head, here.'

'Mhmm.' Suzy's facial expression invited Michael to say a little more.

'He's easy to get caught up in analysing. I mean, he gives me a lot to think about. And he tells me that he has spent much of his life thinking about things, replaying events and how he responded, thinking about other ways of acting or what else he might have said. A lot of time in his head.'

'Does he put you in your head?'

'I have to guard against it.'

'So you are aware of the temptation?'

'Yes, I've had to refocus myself. I've also found myself wondering about his past. He hasn't said much about his childhood, but I have this strong sense that something may have happened, over and above the apparent lack of affection.'

'OK, we can look at that, but let's not stray from the focus here. Where are your feelings? What are your feelings? We can come back to the speculations.'

While the person-centred supervisor will wish to be non-directive and stay with what the supervisee is bringing, there may be occasions when he or she will deem it necessary to hold the supervisee on a particular issue or focus that has arisen. It could be that if the supervisor, in this example, had allowed Michael to develop his speculations then the same insights would eventually be reached, but by a different route and with the supervisee experiencing a different journey in which his own process is much more present and central to the supervision work.

Perhaps the supervisor is overly caught up in her need to hear Michael's feelings and this is stopping her from hearing Michael's speculative ideas as to what may have happened in the past. The supervisor's last comments may be an example of the supervisor living out something of the client's process in that it could leave Michael feeling unheard as he is basically told not to talk about what has become present for him.

The person-centred counsellor and supervisor will place a great deal of emphasis on seeing congruence, and of generating an understanding of where it seems to be lacking. What could be happening here is that incongruence has become present in the supervision relationship – either through Michael not realising he is not expressing his feelings when he thinks that he is, and/or through Suzy for some reason not being able to hear Michael's feelings that perhaps he is connected with and expressing. What will be important is that supervisor and supervisee take responsibility for their parts in this process.

'Well, I feel the speculation is important. I do think that as well as Peter not getting much affection from his mother – indeed, she was very critical and continues to undermine him – that maybe something else happened as well, and that links to his struggle to ask for things for himself – highlighted when he could not ask for a drink of water in the session, something that made a deep impression on him.' Michael had noted that he really needed to say that, but somehow it had seemed an effort. He voiced this, and continued by then saying that he thought maybe they were in some way living out something of the dynamic that Peter experiences.

Suzy asked Michael how it was leaving him feeling, and he said that it seemed like he was being criticised, that his need to speculate wasn't being honoured. She took on board what Michael was saying. 'Hmm, seems like we are parallel processing here, living out a similar dynamic. But I don't want to slip into theoretical reflection when there is still a process running between us.'

'No, neither do I, save that for later. I'm irritated that I was directed away from speculation about something that I feel is quite important. I do sense something significant happened and I do want to explore that.'

'And I was asking about your feelings, and it seems that what has emerged is a strong set of feelings linked to feeling irritated by my response.' Suzy thought for a moment. 'So, you wanted to speculate and not focus on your feelings just now, and now I'm seeking to speculate on what is happening between us but you have feelings to express, so a sudden flip-over has occurred as well.'

'It all happened so fast. Yes, we've reversed, like a switch of polarity. What was happening?'

Suzy smiled. 'You know, part of me wants to explore the feelings around all of this, and another part wants to think about it theoretically, and that's exactly the split we're struggling with.'

'OK, so maybe this head/heart split is significant, and the fact that it moves around. Could it help us understand Peter's process and the way he relates to his mother? And saying that, I'm aware of turning it back towards speculation again.'

'It seems to be flowing back and forward here, and I wonder how much your client, Peter, is also subject to that fluidity, and maybe his mother as well. I mean, I just wonder because sometimes people can be very fluid, can switch very quickly, and if a parent does that to a child, first of all they learn that as a way of being, but they initially find themselves confused, struggling to keep up, to make sense of what is happening. I don't want to stereotype, and yet this is what I'm doing, because I know how incongruent some parents can be, one moment being all nice to a child, the next being hyper-critical.'

'Not sure of the nice part, Peter hasn't really talked about that. But certainly the critical aspect is there. I guess he tries to be nice, well, he's said about wanting to feel affection.' Michael was suddenly back in his own feelings.

'You've shifted.' Suzy was aware of the change in Michael's expression.

'Yes, it's his craving affection – I think I'd put it as strong as that, but it's also kept down as well, I guess. He so wants to feel loved, cared for, and he wants that from his mum, but she's not offering it. He's been out with a woman from work, I'm not sure how much relational experience he has had, but maybe that's timely. But, my God, if it ever develops his mother is likely to react. I wouldn't want to be Peter's girlfriend if it develops.'

'I kind of think she might experience a really hard time, though perhaps a mixture of nice and nasty maybe.'

Michael was taking a deep breath and shaking his head. He was tight-lipped as he thought of Peter, of the emotion he had expressed in relation to the loss of his father, so much sensitivity and emotion, and somewhere deep within him a little boy crying out for love. And at the same time, a man crying out for independence.

So, Peter has developed a structure of self to cope with the reactions of his parents. His father was ineffectual in many ways but provided Peter with a male role model. So it is likely that within him he has constructed a discrete sense of self, a configuration or part as described previously, patterned on his father.

Peter will very likely also have a configuration that will be linked to his need for love and affection, a bereft sense of self, although it will be for him to acknowledge and define what this is in his own words. It is not for the therapist to try to name or define the 'parts' that are present within a client. There is also the part of him wanting his independence, wanting to assert his individuality and break free of the influence of his mother. Another part of himself may well carry the belief that he is deserving of criticism, that he was and is 'not good enough', an area within his structure of self where low self-esteem is focused. There will no doubt be other 'parts' or 'configurations' as well, each contributing to the personhood that is Peter.

Person-centred therapy offers an opportunity for the parts to emerge and to be experienced and understood, to be perhaps redefined or maybe regenerated from the standpoint of Peter the adult. The therapeutic process should lead to the possibility of greater integration and congruence within his self-structure and his experience of himself. The parts may emerge distinct from each other, or Peter may simply move through them without necessarily thinking of them or experiencing them in this way.

'I'm so aware of the struggle that Peter faces. I'm also thinking back to my own experience which is such a contrast to Peter, and maybe that makes it more acute for me, trying to imagine what it must have been like for him. I wonder if he ever felt wanted, and if he didn't why did it happen? Why was he rejected, if that's what happened?' He paused. 'So many questions and speculations, and yet they can take me away from the reality of the experience of being in therapeutic relationship with Peter. We felt – I felt – really close that last session and I am sure that something is going to emerge, or happen. He's feeling more on edge, more unaccepting of his mother.'

Suzy nodded slowly; her thoughts had moved to wondering about Michael's needs as he sat with Peter. But she also wanted to acknowledge hearing what he had just said. 'A lot of closeness, you felt it in that last session. I'm wondering what will help you stay close?'

Michael stopped to think. A good question, he thought to himself. What do I need? Can I stay with him? What will I be asked to stay with? He didn't know. But he knew it was powerful. The kind of relationship issue that Peter was working on was such a fundamental one to the human experience. Some would probably describe it in archetypal terms. 'No doubt Freud would have had a lot to say on the matter! Not that I have any sense of some Oedipal urge with Peter wanting to kill his father to have sex with his mother – though having said that, in a way the father did not stand up for Peter to help him get more affection, and maybe for other reasons he might have harboured a wish to see him dead. But that's total speculation and, well, not what I'm experiencing from Peter. He clearly loved his father, but that doesn't mean he didn't have other feelings too.' Michael blew out a breath. 'It can get so complicated once you start and I'm not sure that's helpful just at the moment. We don't know what happened, other than that Peter did not get the affection he wanted, needed. And he's now stuck in an unhealthy relationship with his mother, full of all kinds of feelings and thoughts going back to his earliest years, grieving for his father and coming to me to try to help himself get a fresh start in life.' Michael felt overwhelmed, and Suzy was also struck by the immensity of it all.

'What do *you* need, Michael?'

Michael stuck out his lower lip as he wrestled with the question. And yet he knew he didn't have to wrestle with it because the answer was present immediately. He needed what Peter needed. He needed to feel warmth and caring, sensitivity and respect, as he sought to describe his encounters with Peter. He needed to have the human responses reinforced. He also felt that he had to avoid being too much in his head speculating and theorising. He expressed this, and then continued. 'I need simplicity here. I need to bring my human self, my human reactions, into my relationship with you. I need to be able to allow myself to be affected deeply by Peter, and I feel that is happening, and I must not close down. I don't think I will, but I have to make sure. I have to be open. I need to use supervision to maintain my openness and sensitivity.'

Suzy nodded; she didn't feel she had anything to add to what Michael was asking for.

Michael continued. 'I may go into speculation and, yes, I do want a theoretical appreciation of the process, but I need to be sure I can sit with Peter, with whatever emerges. He must have so much locked up inside himself. It's not going to be a short process, is it?'

'Maybe not, up to Peter, I guess. We don't know how far he will want to take this. If he tries to make changes in his life, the parts of himself that don't want to change – and they'll exist somewhere – are bound to fight back and may seek to sabotage the therapy, perhaps. But it brings us back into speculation again.'

'Hmm. It might be a slow process, with a lot of twists and turns.'

'And it may be a series of sudden shifts, each separated by lengthy periods where little seems to happen.'

Michael could feel that while he had a sense of how overwhelming it was, he also felt a sense of privilege to be involved in working with Peter at this critical time in his life. He voiced this and added that he hoped that he could be good for him, that he could contribute effectively in creating the therapeutic climate that would help Peter and allow the actualising tendency within him to move him towards resolving the incongruencies and negative conditioning that had played a major part in his development. The supervision session drew to a close. Michael left feeling that while the supervision session had ranged across a variety of issues, and had seemingly provided a vehicle for living out some of the dynamics that were present for his client in what must appear from the outside as being in a rather haphazard way, it also felt like he had done some useful work. He felt a little less knotted – he hadn't thought of it that way before, but yes, that image did seem to fit. It was like he had loosened something, or at least felt looser inside. Yet he was also focused too, and determined to help Peter to gain as much as he could from therapy.

He thought about goals. Person-centred working is a non-directive approach, and yet he had to be honest and say that, yes, he had a goal. He wanted Peter to discover his potential, claim his identity as an individual, as a man. He hoped that he could resolve his relationship with his mother in some mutually productive way. Whether that was possible, he did not know. And it might not be what Peter needed, or maybe it was. Back to the speculation. It frustrated him.

His thoughts stayed with Peter throughout his journey home to his partner who had prepared a meal for them. Marty was good for him, always seemed so sensitive and able to calm him down when things got on top of him. He was smiling by the time he'd arrived. He'd been so fortunate, his parents had been so accepting of him when he had come out and told them he was gay. Initially they'd been uneasy, unconvinced, and, yes, he'd had difficult times, struggling with his feelings and his sexuality, experimenting with different relationships, but he had settled into the relationship with Marty and his parents really liked him. He was suddenly very grateful. How different it could have been – his thoughts went to Peter. He opened the door to the flat with a sense of gratitude and appreciation, and made a mental note to call his mother that evening, to say 'hi' and 'I love you'.

CHAPTER 4

Counselling session 5: discomfort within the therapeutic relationship

29 September

Peter seemed withdrawn. He looked like he'd had a tough week. Michael enquired
   as to how he was.
'I told her.'
Michael guessed that Peter was referring to his mother.
'Mhmm, must have taken a lot of courage.' Michael wanted to convey an apprecia-
   tion of how difficult it must have been, although Peter hadn't actually said that.

> It might seem like a therapeutically helpful response, but as in this instance
> it is clear that Michael's perception does not match Peter's experience.
> Maybe he might have just confirmed who he had spoken to, for instance,
> 'Your mother?' What might be clear from Michael's response is his own
> sense that for him it would be brave to say this to Peter's mother if he was
> Peter. But he isn't.

'Actually, no. After our last session I was determined. And I just out and said it
   when I got back. Told her I was seeing a counsellor and talking things through,
   and thinking about my life and where it was going.'
'Determined and out and told her.'
Peter nodded as he sat back in the chair.
Michael was bursting to enquire what happened, but he bit it back, giving Peter
   time to say what he wanted to say and at his own pace.
Peter was pursing his lips. 'Didn't go down too well. "You don't need to see someone like that, telling them all about yourself." She just didn't want to know.
   I tried to reason with her, tried to calmly tell her I needed time and space to
   myself. Would she have it? Like hell. It was a frosty atmosphere the rest of the
   evening.' He was shaking his head. 'Then, next morning, it was like nothing

had happened. She'd cooked my breakfast and was fine, nice as anyone could be. She can be like that, you know, and I foolishly believed that she had accepted it. I should know better, but I always hope that when she's like that, well, that it's genuine and will stick, but it never does. And it didn't.' He paused again.

'So she was nice and you hoped that she would stay that way though from experience you knew it wasn't likely.'

'Little comments, you know, and wanting to know what I was saying. Just went on over the next few days. What was I talking about? Was I talking about her? What did I need to talk to a stranger about? Keep it in the family. Didn't have counselling when she was younger – I wanted to say "more's the pity", but didn't, would have just thrown fuel on the fire. Wouldn't have achieved anything, but I sure felt it.'

'Mhmm.'

A weak response. It would have been more therapeutically helpful to have said something like, 'You sure felt like saying "more's the pity".' It would have captured the intensity as well as the focus.

'I told her I'd talked about dad and that I had got upset and emotional. She immediately cut in and said, "Serves you right, stirring yourself up over it."'

Michael was looking at the expression on Peter's face. He looked absolutely raging.

'You reacted? You look bloody angry.'

'I was, but I didn't say anything.' Peter looked sad as he tightened his jaw.

'You didn't say anything to her but you felt like it.'

'What's the point? She's not going to change, nothing I say will make a difference. She doesn't listen, not interested in listening. As far as she is concerned everything is fine, doesn't want anything to disturb her world.' There was a sarcastic edge to Peter's voice, and this was new to Michael.

'Mhmm, that's how it seems, what's the point, she won't change.' He reflected back the tone of voice.

'This morning, "So I suppose you're going to see this counsellor again." I didn't say anything at first. She persisted. Made me more determined to keep coming. This is the one place where I feel listened to.' Peter closed his eyes. 'Apart from work, it is somewhere I can get away from her. Apart from seeing Melanie – we've been out again.' Michael noted that Peter's face visibly brightened as he mentioned her name, though he also looked a little embarrassed too.

'So, your mother was critical but it leaves you more determined. Having space to feel listened to, and Melanie's important as well.'

'Yes, we went to a concert – sort of 1960s show. It was good, we enjoyed ourselves, going out again on Friday.'

'Sounds great.' Michael left Peter with his feelings; he clearly had had a good time and he was pleased that those feelings could also be brought into the therapeutic environment – such a contrast to what else Peter was experiencing.

'Yes, feels strange. I mean, I don't know, just feel strange.'

'Feels strange?' Michael invited Peter to say a little more.

'How I feel. I mean, it feels good being with her. I feel kind of free somehow, like I've kind of lost weight. It's like stepping out of one world into another. It feels so good.'

'Quite a contrast, and it leaves you feeling kind of free and it feels good.' Michael was aware that he was smiling and nodding slightly. He sat back in his chair, unaware that he had previously moved forward.

'Yes.' Peter felt good as he thought about it. There was something about Melanie. He'd got to know her a little more now and, yes, he felt different.

Note the speed at which Peter has changed, both in his demeanour and his focus. Bringing his experience of being with Melanie into the session has produced a clear shift. It might be experienced by the counsellor as though he was desperately grasping at something. Through this new relationship it seems that Peter is engaging with feelings, and perhaps aspects of himself, that were previously unknown. Whatever happens in the relationship it has offered Peter an experience, a glimpse of another possibility for himself. It is powerful. Time will tell the true ramifications of this experience.

Michael was aware that while Peter was speaking of feeling lighter, and freer, in fact his shoulders looked tight and raised. Lot of tension in his body, he thought to himself. Michael consciously dropped his own shoulders.

Peter had noticed Michael's movement and it brought his own shoulders to his attention, and the fact that they felt tense. He sat forward a little and stretched his arms back to free them off. 'Too long in front of the computer. Should get up more often, move around, free myself off, but I forget.'

Michael appears to drop his shoulders consciously in response to his perception of the tightness in Peter's body. He has stepped out of being person-centred and has been directive, with Peter now focused on the tension in his body. Perhaps Michael was experiencing tension in his own body but there is not ownership of this in the therapeutic exchange.

'Easily done. We carry a lot of stress in the shoulders.'

'Yeah. I feel it at home. I can feel it as I walk up the path some evenings – depends what my day has been like at work, but I really notice it after I've been with Melanie. I can feel myself tensing up. I'm realising how much I want to get rid of it.'

'Get rid of that tension.' Michael kept his response to the point, not wanting to interrupt the flow.

Peter sat quietly. He suddenly took a deep breath. 'I had this dream. I was driving along a road, it was kind of dark, and I come up to a kind of junction, and I've got to decide which way to go.'

'Mhmm.'

'It was like a kind of fork in the road, or rather, more like the road I was on kind of continued to the left and went down and sort of seemed to be darker somehow. Had a sense that it wasn't really going anywhere although I kind of felt I knew it, that it was sort of familiar somehow. And then there's a road on the right, and that seemed to be heading up a hill, at least some kind of incline, and there seemed to be a village ahead, there were lights in the distance. It wasn't like it was a junction I kind of knew, I mean, I couldn't think of it as somewhere I'd been, and yet somehow I did know the dark road on the left, like I'd been down it, but didn't want to go down it again.'

'Sounds powerful – the junction, the familiar road to the left that you sensed went nowhere, and the one on the right, towards lights from a village.' Michael felt the urge to speculate to himself as to the meaning but pushed it aside. He wanted to hear what Peter had to say, what it meant to him.

The person-centred counsellor is not going to interpret dreams. He or she will listen to what a client has experienced and, if the client has interpreted them, listen to what they have to say. However, the symbolism of dreams is linked to the experience of the dreamer. An example of this could be that a client talks of, let us say, the image of a lion. Normally, this might be seen as symbolising strength, courage, maybe something to fear. However, the client may actually associate the image of a lion with feelings connected to the toy lion they had as a child, something that was a focus for a great deal of love and affection, or something precious that perhaps they lost at some point in their lives.

By allowing the client to make their own associations they are not only more likely to accurately understand what meaning the dream may have for them, but also more accurately integrate both the dream and its meaning into their awareness. Sometimes dreams are external reflections of inner processes. Engaging with the dream can help to integrate experiences that may have become dissociated or feel out of reach.

'My life's at a crossroads, Michael, and I've got to decide which way to go. It's like I've been travelling along this road and, well, I could carry straight on, but that doesn't seem to go anywhere. And there's a road going off to the right and that kind of appeals, but it's sort of unknown. And I've pulled up and I'm trying to decide which way to go. I haven't got a map, and I'm low on fuel.'

'Mhmm, Sounds quite tense.'

'I woke up in the middle of the night, feeling really anxious. Seemed to feel unable to decide which way to go, and it felt so important to make a decision. I was sweating, my stomach was churning, my throat was dry. I felt really disturbed by it. It was so vivid, so real.'

'Sounds like it made a huge impact on you.' Michael kept his response non-specific, though with the intention of helping Peter stay with the effect it had had on him.

Peter was taking a deep breath. Yes, it had made a deep impact. It had somehow been unsettling. Yet it had been so vivid, so present for him. 'I had to decide which way to go, but I couldn't.'

'Mhmm. Which way to go . . .'

'. . . and I didn't know although I mean I do know, but in the dream I didn't. It was like I did but I didn't.'

'Like you did know which way to go but at the same time you didn't?'

Peter nodded. 'I knew I had to take that road to the right, and yet somehow it felt like I couldn't, and yet I had to, and then I woke up. I was really affected by it.'

Michael couldn't help but think what a simple and yet so timely a dream, given what Peter had said about telling his mother about the counselling. It almost felt like it was a natural development of the process that was underway for him. 'Yes, as you tell me I can sense the importance of it for you.' Michael could see by the expression on Peter's face just how the dream had impacted on him. He was somehow looking very intense. He wasn't sure that he had seen Peter look quite like that before. 'I sense it to have been – and it still is – quite an intense experience.'

'Had to make a choice, knew which way I had to go, but couldn't, not in the dream. Kept looking at the map, filled with a sense of not knowing . . . of just not knowing.' Peter could feel himself reconnecting with the dream experience. There was some vividness still present for him. And as he thought about it, he recalled something else, and he was surprised that he had forgotten to mention it. The voice of his father telling him it was OK, that he should keep going, no need to stop, keep going. As he remembered this he felt himself shiver.

Michael noticed the physical reaction. 'Something else?'

'My father's voice.'

'Just now or in the dream?'

'In the dream, urging me to continue, "Don't stop, keep going, it's OK, keep going" and though I heard him I still stopped, hesitated and then couldn't get going again.'

'Mhmm, so in spite of his urging you stopped, and then couldn't move on.'

Peter tightened his lips. 'Stuck, sums it up.'

Michael nodded. 'That was how you felt, sitting there.' Michael has kept the focus on the dream; however, Peter may have shifted with his last comment back into his present.

The dream is, of course, open to interpretation, but Michael has maintained a person-centred attitude by not imposing an interpretation. This may mean that the dream is not explored as much as it might otherwise have been, but that is OK. The client knows if they feel that the dream is pressing enough for further exploration. It is for the counsellor to offer the therapeutic environment such that the client feels able to undertake this exploration should they so wish to. The counsellor trusts the therapeutic value of this process of relationship building, and the process within the client that enables them to know what they feel capable of addressing, and in what manner.

Trusting the process of the client and of the therapeutic relationship is at the heart of person-centred therapy. Thorne (1996, p. 139) writes that 'there is trust in the innate resourcefulness of human beings, given the right conditions, to find their own way through life. There is trust that the direction thus found will be positive and creative. There is trust, too, that the process between counsellor and client will in itself provide the primary context of safety and nurture in which the client can face the pain of alienation from his or her true self and move towards a more integrated way of being.'

'Not just there, but here, now, in life.' Peter shook his head. He knew he had to change, to move on, to break free. He felt tears in his eyes and a lump in his throat as he thought about his father. 'He was so clear, so close.' He dropped his head, tightening his lips once again. He took another deep breath and let the air out slowly. His father, he thought, he'd never got away – only to the grave. He began to speculate, finding himself wondering how much of a life his father had really had. He felt sadness for him, then it moved and he could feel sadness for his mother too. Between them both they had, perhaps, wasted an opportunity for something better, perhaps something more loving.

Michael sat in the silence. It did not feel forced or uncomfortable. He guessed Peter was thinking about things and he allowed him to stay with his process.

Peter was experiencing images of his parents together – often arguing. He tried to think of a time when they had seemed happy together. He was shocked to realise that he couldn't think of one. He had been looking down and he suddenly remembered where he was – not that he'd really forgotten, but his thoughts, his memories had momentarily taken over. He looked up, and felt he should say something.

'You looked deep in thought.'

'Trying to think of happy times with my parents, or rather, between them.' He paused, shaking his head. 'I couldn't.' He felt the wave of sadness again.

'Hmm.' Michael was taking a deep breath himself. 'No memories of happy times.'

Michael has emphasised that what is not present are the memories. Peter has not necessarily said that there were no happy times, simply that he cannot recall any. Michael's empathic response holds Peter in the experience of what is lacking in his memory, which is what he had communicated to Michael.

Peter realised that he wished he did have memories of his parents getting on, and he was sure there must have been times – maybe when he was much younger – when things were better between them. He hoped so, but it was unsettling not to know, not to be sure, not to have any clear memories. It somehow felt empty, dry – no, not so much dry, more barren, that was a better word for it. He could still feel the sadness that was present within him. He didn't want to cry, it wasn't affecting him quite like that. But he knew that the emptiness he felt was deep and went back a long way. He sat in silence – outwardly at least. Inside he wasn't silence, he was rather lost in his sense of emptiness, a place that somehow felt safe, felt familiar, felt OK, and yet not OK as well. It was an uncomfortable place but he was used to it.

Michael sat and kept his focus on Peter, holding in his mind the comments Peter had been making and being aware of his feeling for Peter in his struggle ... He was about to think to himself in terms of Peter's *struggle to*, but realised he did not know what Peter was struggling towards. The dream was a representation of a journey, of choice, of a decision to be made, but where it would lead him, what the struggle was towards, he did not know. Greater freedom and independence? Fuller sense of himself and his potential as a person? Set aside the sense of being a son and become the man?

Michael's thoughts wandered and he thought of Peter as a seed planted in the ground. He thought of the core conditions, of the warm acceptance, the empathic responding and the genuine presence that he sought to bring into the therapeutic relationship as being representative of warmth, light and water being given to that seed, to help it germinate, or to strengthen the roots and shoot that were developing. He didn't know what the seed would grow into. He wasn't much of a gardener anyway. The image had become more distinct for Michael. Yes, a seed, but what will it grow into?

> The person-centred therapist offers the climate of relationship that encourages growth, emergence, the thrust of the actualising tendency. But what will emerge is unknown. The therapist working from a theoretical and experiential base that is person-centred will not try to make the client become this or grow towards or into that. The potential is contained within the client, or symbolically within the seed alluded to above.

Michael brought his attention back, and he was aware that Peter was looking at him. 'You look as though you drifted off.'

'I was thinking about you, what you had said, and trying to be open to what I was experiencing. My thoughts then went to an image, to that of a seed, and how given the right climate it will germinate and grow. Just thinking of counselling as providing such a climate for people to grow.' Michael was not at ease with what he had said. He had made it general, but what he had been experiencing was specific and focused on Peter. He therefore continued in order to preserve his genuineness and transparency. 'I was thinking specifically of you, and realising how you will grow, change, in your own way through therapy – what the seed, that is you, will develop into.'

Listening to Michael speak felt good. It felt like he really cared, that he was giving his thoughts to wonder about how he, Peter, might change. It generated within Peter a sense that someone cared, and yet that also seemed really hard to accept.

'Right.' He spoke quite abruptly. He wasn't feeling abrupt, but that was how he spoke.

Michael sensed a change of atmosphere between them; he wasn't sure what it was about. What Peter had said didn't feel right, even though that was the word he had used. There was some kind of mis-match, and he wasn't sure how to respond. He felt himself losing his spontaneity, he was thinking about it, about his reaction, about what he was experiencing within himself. He'd lost connection with Peter. He felt he needed to say something but wasn't sure what. He could feel the hesitancy as he thought about what to say.

'I don't know quite what to say, Peter, I feel like something just happened then and I'm not sure what it was, or is that's happening.'

Michael is aware of hesitancy; he is struggling to find words. Although he has not identified it, he may be experiencing anxiety to some degree. It could be indicative of something incongruent emerging within himself, but perhaps triggered by Peter. He senses something isn't right.

Peter has entered an incongruent state. While he senses that he is being cared for he is finding it hard to accept, and some other aspect of himself, some other 'part', has cut in with the abrupt 'right' that perhaps is carrying a disbelieving tone. He may have body language giving one signal, but a tone of voice giving another. Michael ends up confused. It is vital that he strives to stay with his reaction and his own transparency. He has rightly identified the moment and conveyed his sense of something happening.

Peter felt suddenly uncomfortable, and quite strongly so. He had liked feeling cared for, that Michael had been thinking about him and the idea that he would grow as from a seed into something, or someone, through therapy. He wasn't sure quite what Michael was talking about. He was confused.

'What do you mean?'

Michael realised that the focus had shifted to himself and that was not his intention, and yet he needed to be transparent and trust that his wrestling with what was present for him would have therapeutic value for Peter and contribute to the transparency of their relationship.

'After I said about what I was thinking about, what effect therapy might have for you, your response felt to me – and it is my experience – rather abrupt. And yet I wasn't experiencing you up until that moment as being abrupt; rather it felt like we were connected, you were listening to what I was saying.'

Peter felt an instinct to take a deep breath – he acted upon it. He didn't feel abrupt, felt a bit confused, not sure what Michael was getting at. 'I don't know what you mean. Apart from feeling strange talking like this, I feel OK. I heard what you said.' He shrugged.

Michael nodded slowly, not sure himself, and yet also feeling sure that something had happened. But he recognised that if Peter was not experiencing anything significant then perhaps he should let it go and explore it himself in super-vision. Maybe he was being over-sensitive and, if so, he needed to explore why. If not, and something had happened, maybe he needed to acknowledge it and allow it to rest, accepting that if something was important for Peter's process – and perhaps for their therapeutic process – then it might arise again. He didn't want to speculate too much or start drawing conclusions. Accept and move on. Focus back on Peter.

'Mhmm. Yes, kind of made you feel strange hearing me talking like that.' Michael paused. He decided not to put down his experience, or make some excuse for himself, both of which would be defensive and he didn't actually feel he had anything to defend. He felt he had been open in the moment. He was aware of his own hesitancy and felt sure something significant had happened, but he wasn't going to push it. He respected Peter's own process and that he needed to work with him to allow anything to emerge when the time was right. Maybe something had emerged and, if this was the case, Peter was choosing not to see it, or maybe part of him was stopping him from seeing it. Michael knew specu-lation could be endless – he wasn't here to speculate. As a person-centred counsellor he needed to stay with his client – he'd discuss it in supervision.

'Yes. Unsettled me.'

'Still feeling unsettled?'

'Not so much. But wondering what it was all about.'

'I'm not sure whether you want to continue to focus on this – and I'm aware that we haven't much time left in the session. And having said that I also don't want to lose sight of what you have just said – that you are wondering what it was all about.'

'I think I need to think about it, Michael. I kind of trust you and, well, if something made a kind of impact on you, well, then maybe I need to, I don't know, look at it?'

'And I want to respond by saying that I'm wondering now whether, if this is the case, whether it is because you want to look at it, or you feel you ought to look at it.'

Michael felt uncomfortable again. He was stepping out of his person-centred attitude.

Michael could have empathised in a simple and straightforward manner: 'You kind of wonder if you need to look at it.' This may have been more ther-apeutically valuable; however, the point about the impact of Peter's trust of Michael leaving him experiencing a need to look at it gets lost.

'Got enough things I ought to do in my life.' Peter paused; he was hesitating. He was feeling somewhat pissed off, but he wasn't sure why, with whom or with what. He took another deep breath, tightening his lips as he did so. He felt a yawn coming on. And an urge to stretch. 'I'm really not sure. I'm feeling tired and think maybe I need to call it a day.'

Michael stayed with him, seeking an empathic response. He nodded. 'Feel ready
to stop, yeah, tiring.'

Peter nodded. His eyes felt heavy all of a sudden.

The time was nearly up and the session drew to a close. Michael made a point of
checking that Peter was OK, feeling concerned that it was all very abrupt – and
he was aware that this 'abruptness' seemed somehow to be a distinguishing
feature of some aspect of Peter that was emerging. He knew that with the session ending – and he was not going to run over time – he needed a break
before his next client and recognised his duty to that next client. He also recognised within himself an acceptance that for whatever reason Peter needed to be
how he was – that a process was running for him and he wanted to not get in
the way of it. So having checked that Peter was OK, the session ended.

Peter left and was actually feeling quite anxious. His heart was pounding a little,
but he really knew he needed to leave, and he was glad the session had ended.
It wasn't that he felt a need to avoid talking about anything, there was nothing
dramatic in his head, but he just felt the need to get out, get some air and
head off. It was later that evening, when he was sitting on the bed in his
room just before retiring, that he suddenly burst into tears. He didn't know
why. He finally slept but more from the tiredness of crying into his pillow. The
only thought that was with him was a sense of his life passing by – and an
overwhelming feeling, of suddenly feeling very alone. He'd felt alone before,
but never quite like that. He had a very restless night.

Clearly a lot is going on for Peter in terms of his inner process, and it is interesting that following on from the emergence of his incongruence concerning
his abruptness there now follows a feeling of tiredness that induces an end
to the session. Yes, the client has every right to feel tired and feel he needs to
leave. The person-centred counsellor will wish to convey warm acceptance
of the client's need and his intention to act upon it. As a result the client, and
importantly the parts of the client that are inducing the client's experience
and behaviour, are going to feel warmly accepted.

   This may sound complicated. But what it means is that the part of Peter
that finds it hard to feel warmth is itself now being offered warm acceptance,
and the part that seeks to end the session by inducing tiredness is also being
heard and allowed to have its needs met without questioning. While some
might argue it is collusion, I would suggest that what is happening is that
these parts of Peter's structure of self are being allowed to manifest within
the therapeutic relationship, and it is hoped that this will continue, and that
they will feel it is a safe place and perhaps, in time, the reasons for which
they were generated will also emerge.

   It is highly likely that it is the same part that is emerging, a part that does
not want, or is not used or is unable, to hear that Michael is genuinely interested in Peter and perceives his potential to grow and develop. Its final

attempt to stop this experience is to induce tiredness, get the session ended and get away from the threat that Michael's congruence and warmth are being experienced as.

Counselling session 6: cancelled appointment

6 October

Peter cancelled the next appointment, carefully phoning at a time when he expected to reach the answer machine. He really did not want to attend, well, he had mixed feelings but he was unsettled by that last session and really did not want to go. He had also had a busy week at work, taking on extra tasks which, in reality, he knew would eat into his evenings and give him an excuse for not attending. He had phoned to say that he was cancelling because of work. He somehow felt that that was OK, although at heart he knew it was an excuse. He didn't want to go. He didn't feel ready to face the discomfort that last session had aroused in him.

He busied himself, working into the evening, and exhausting himself. He slept each night, but it wasn't very restful, well, not for most of the nights. The dream repeated itself on a couple of occasions, though with the addition of his mother, standing at the fork in the roads, telling him not to listen to his father. It left him confused.

His work wasn't up to its usual standards. He made mistakes, errors that he would normally have picked up. He found himself more irritable, not just with himself but with others – and at home. He lost touch with the thought of leaving; rather he just spent time on his own. He worked on his own not having much time for anyone else, and he spent a lot of time alone at home – often in front of his computer. He didn't want to think, he didn't want to feel.

Michael was given the message that Peter had cancelled, and that there had been no mention of whether he wanted another appointment. Michael wanted to allow Peter the space that he clearly was asking for, and yet he also knew he needed to check out whether Peter planned to continue and, if not, how they might process an ending if that was what Peter wished for. He decided to phone after the appointment, when Peter would have passed through his own reactions to not attending, and then discuss the next step. Peter had phoned early on the Monday, the appointment being for the Tuesday evening. He let Wednesday pass in case Peter might initiate a call, but he did not. Michael meanwhile was pondering his response – phone or write?

He decided to write; it was less invasive and while it meant uncertainty would remain – he would still not know for definite whether Peter wanted to continue or would attend the next appointment – he felt that as the counsellor he should bear that uncertainty and allow Peter his time to think, reflect, make whatever choice he needed to make. Michael knew that his letter would need to be sensitively written, from the heart and to the point.

Dear Peter

Sorry you were unable to make it to your counselling session this week, but thanks very much for calling to let me know. It must be a busy week for you with your increased workload.

I realise I am making an assumption that you would want another appointment. I can see you next Tuesday at 6.00pm as usual. If you do not expect to attend, can you call me? Perhaps we can discuss it, if that is what you would like.

Counselling is not always an easy process, and we can have doubts about it. Sometimes it helps to talk these through.

Warm regards

Michael

Michael spent a while pondering whether to include the last sentence. He didn't want to make and convey an assumption, and yet he felt very strongly that it was more than a work issue. He often found it a dilemma what to say in these cases. He didn't like the idea of a form letter to send to every client – he wanted it personal, he wanted to be able to convey something of himself in what he wrote. He wrote the letter on the Wednesday evening when Peter would have attended. It also felt important to him to have Peter in his mind – and his heart – at the time of their session. He strongly believed that this was somehow a valuable attitude. Yes, he wanted to hold Peter in his thoughts. He felt that Peter would probably be thinking of the session he was missing, though he had no idea what form that thought would take. So he sat quietly holding Peter in his thoughts, the impression that he had made and the issues that had been presented. That word – abruptness – kept coming back to him. He trusted that it had significance though he did not know why.

Peter received the letter on the Friday when he got home from work. He hadn't phoned for another appointment – he really did not know what to do. He felt sorry now that he had cancelled – or, rather, that he had lied about work. He knew he had deliberately made himself busy. He wasn't fooling himself. But the interesting thing was that he made a point of coming home that Tuesday at the time that he would have done had he gone to the counselling – wanted his mother to think that that was where he had been.

He put the letter down. Somehow he knew he had to go back. He had calmed down since the last weekend. He knew he wasn't totally comfortable with the idea, but something was nagging inside him not to give up. He couldn't really define what it was. It wasn't a voice exactly, and it was kind of indistinct, and yet it was there – subtle and yet somehow not so subtle. Persistent. He decided he'd think about it and sat down to eat.

It pre-occupied his thoughts. His mother was talking – telling him something inconsequential about her day. He wasn't interested – well, he rarely was these days, but this time it was different. His thoughts were pre-occupied. Should he phone now, or later? Should he go to see Michael again, or not? Did he know what was best for him? What would his father say? He knew what his mother would say. The dream was in his mind again.

He finished eating and decided he'd listen to some music. He wasn't sure what to listen to. He felt he wanted something calm and soothing, but he got bored with it. Rather he realised he wanted something with power, something to blast his thoughts out of his head – but Meat Loaf's 'Bat Out of Hell' wasn't achieving that either. However, it did leave him thinking . . . as he heard the words:

I know that I'm damned if I never get out
And maybe I'm damned if I do
But with every beat I've got left in my heart
You know I'd never be damned with you.

He thought of Melanie. He felt sad . . . the song was continuing.

But if I've got to be damned you know I want to be damned . . . ,
      got to be damned you know I want to be damned . . . ,
      got to be damned you know I want to be damned . . . ,
   dancing through the night, dancing through the night, dancing through
the night with you. (Steinman, 1993)

He thought of that 60s evening. Dancing through the night with you, with Melanie. He smiled. The song was still continuing. He heard the growling motor bike, the guitar solo screamed into his ears . . . Something happened, something screamed back. There were tears in his eyes and goosebumps up his back, his neck and down the backs of his arms. He felt a surge of energy. Shit, I've got to get out, got to get out, like . . . like . . . like a *bat out of hell*. He was standing up, his fists and jaw clenched, yes, he knew he had to get out, he had to. He needed to be in touch with what he was feeling. He played the song again. Yes, yes, a bat out of hell – well, the song wasn't really about his situation, but it touched him, fired him, and he knew he must do something. He didn't know what.

His heart was thudding as he knew what he needed to do – call Melanie. He needed to talk, he had to talk. He called her. She was home. He explained he needed to talk – could they meet up, sorry it was short notice, but was she free? How he hoped she was. The reply came back, 'yes'. He felt himself taking a deep breath, and his heart thumped a little more. They agreed a time.

Peter put down the phone. OK – the counselling. He called Michael. No one was in by now so he left a message confirming he would be back the next week, that he would see Michael at the usual time, that he was sorry he'd missed the appointment but that maybe he'd needed to, and would talk about it when he saw him. His heart was still pounding but he felt good. He felt energised, like he'd risen out of his pit. Yeah, he thought, like a bat out of hell.

He got ready to go. As he was about to leave the room, he glanced at the tape player. Went over, took out the tape and put in his pocket. Something for the car. He was smiling as he left the room.

Points for discussion

- What was your reaction to Peter's dream? Did you find yourself interpreting it? What would you have done with this interpretation in the session?
- Evaluate Michael's congruence. Do you feel he is effectively applying the person-centred approach? If so, why? If not, why not?
- What were the key moments in the last session that Peter attended?
- Therapeutic relationship can be uncomfortable. How do you handle discomfort when it arises?
- Without further reference to the letter in the text, write your own letter to Peter and then contrast this with Michael's. Reflect on the reasons for similarities and differences.
- Pick out two key issues that you would want to take to supervision from what has occurred.
- Write counselling notes for the two sessions.

CHAPTER 5

Counselling session 7: a memory surfaces, 'Can I have a drink of water?'

13 October

Peter arrived on time; in fact he was a bit early. He had listened to the tape again on the way over. Yes, he was ready to face whatever needed to be faced. He was ready ...

Michael came into the waiting room and Peter was standing looking at some posters on the noticeboard.

'Hi Peter, come on through.'

Peter turned. 'Thanks. Good to see you.'

Michael was struck by the firmness in Peter's voice.

'You too. You sound positive.'

'Yep.' They had reached the counselling room and Peter was sitting down. Michael noticed that there was no hesitancy, made him realise just how hesitant Peter had seemed when he had seen him before. He sat and waited – he didn't have to wait too long.

'Well, it's been quite a couple of weeks. Really bad week after the last session – and I'm really sorry for not coming, really sorry – and yet, well, I'm also glad I didn't.'

'Mhmm.' Michael didn't want to disturb the flow.

'I still don't really know what last time was about, but I know I needed to get away. Anyway, so I didn't come, and then I got your letter and, well, wasn't sure what to do. Left me really with so many conflicting thoughts in my head.' Peter was thinking back to the experience.

Michael took the opportunity of communicating a brief empathic response. 'Head full of conflict ...'

'... and, well, I don't know, just decided I needed to calm down – tried some calming music which didn't work and then, well, not sure why, but decided I needed to blast the thoughts out of my head, you know, just well kind of sand-blast them away, if you know what I mean.'

'Sounds really powerful, sand-blast them away, clean your head out, yes?'

'Yeah, it really was like that. Anyway, I listened to a song by Meat Loaf.'

Didn't mean much to Michael. He was a classical music buff himself; he'd heard of Meat Loaf, and felt himself wanting to smile as he'd wondered whether he was referred to by people as 'Mr Loaf'. He suppressed his smile; it wasn't appropriate to Peter's focus.

'Mhmm. Made an impression?'

Peter was nodding. 'It did. Really took me by surprise, really got hold of me. Wrung some emotions out of me, it really did. But it fired me up too, really fired me up.'

'Fired you up?' Michael was curious as to what Peter meant and he wanted to feel in touch with Peter's process.

'Yeah, yes it did. Some of the words got to me, but then it was the power of the music, I don't know, something happened inside me, something clicked, connected.'

'Mhmm. Powerful, like you connected with something inside you?' Michael was aware that wasn't exactly how Peter had put it.

Peter nodded. He explained what had touched him. 'Touched! Not quite the right word. More like it grabbed hold of me, like it reached deep inside me and grabbed hold and gave me a good shake. It really was like that.'

'Powerful – grabbed hold of, shaken, and something deep.'

'Very deep.' As Peter spoke he was feeling so alive. He was still in touch with whatever it was.

'And it feels . . .?'

'. . . bloody good.'

Michael was struck by Peter's language – he hadn't sworn much in the sessions.

'Mhmm, feels bloody good to be in touch with yourself.'

'Really does. And, well, it was the line "and I know that I'm damned if I never get out, and maybe I'm damned if I do." Yes, it somehow really got to me that. Summed it up. Whatever I do – stay or leave – gonna be damned, feel damned. Either she'll give me hell – well, either way that'll happen. And I can't go on like this. I need out, need space, distance, my own life. Yes, I've got to get out . . .', he hesitated, and then added, 'like a bat out of hell.'

The phrase did not mean anything to Michael. He had not heard of the record. He was struck by the power of the imagery. 'Like a bat out of hell – that's quite a powerful image.'

Peter assumed Michael would know the song, so he didn't explain it, just agreed. 'Yes, but it really sums it up. That's what I need to do, get out of there like a bat out of hell! And I'm going to.'

Even though assumptions are made, even though the counsellor does not know the piece of music being referred to, it does not stop him from empathising effectively with the impact on the client.

Michael was struck by the determination in Peter's voice. 'And you're going to, aren't you?'

Peter nodded. 'Been looking around this week. I've put my name on the council list though there's a huge wait and, well, that's probably not going to happen for a long time. But I don't need that. I've looked at renting. Probably go for a flat somewhere – nothing too big – couple of bedrooms maybe for a bit of extra space. Just think I need space to think, be with myself, give myself time to decide what to do.'

Michael was nodding, appreciating what Peter was saying. He had moved away from home and into a flat himself although his circumstances had been very different. 'So, change, movement, looking for space to be with yourself and think about what to do.'

Peter took a deep breath. It suddenly felt like a big step. But he knew he wanted, no, needed, to make that step. He went on to talk about how he'd called Melanie, how they'd gone out for a drink, how they'd talked – well, how he'd talked and she'd listened. They'd gone out for a drive afterwards and he'd ended up at her place for a coffee. They'd continued to talk – late into the night. It had felt so good. He'd left feeling really energised still – and they'd agreed to meet up again later on the Saturday.

They'd gone out to the cinema, and, well, it had started to get a little physical. They'd kissed in the car afterwards. As Peter described it, '. . . and, yes, just felt so right. We met up again on the Sunday – went for a walk along the river in the afternoon. The sun was shining. Just felt so, so good.' Peter knew he was smiling and it had been a little bit of a hurdle to get over at first, talking about Melanie and his feelings, but now, well, now he was flowing. 'She's helped me to see beyond my little world. Now I can't stop thinking about her. And I feel like I walk around all the time with a smile on my face – people must think I'm weird – and the crazy thing . . . no, wonderful thing is . . . I don't care!' He shrugged his shoulders. He was smiling.

'Sounds wonderful, Peter, I feel really pleased. So much going on, in you, around you . . .'

Peter was aware that over half the session had passed by, and while that felt OK, he also knew he wanted to say something about the last session.

'I'm also aware of what I felt after the last session, and it was real and I kind of feel that there's something I need to sort out in myself as well. And maybe I don't, maybe it's gone, and yet, well, I don't think it has.'

Michael nodded. 'Mhmm. So you want to spend time on the experience from last time? Something left to deal with?'

'Mmm. I think I do. And yet I don't want to lose where I am now.'

'That sounds clear, you want to explore what happened last time, and you don't want it to stop you feeling what you are feeling now.'

Peter took a deep breath – he often did when he felt on edge. He wanted to make sense of what he'd experienced last time – and his reaction to Michael's comments. And needing to get away. But then, well, yes, he thought to himself, needing to get away, he'd certainly been in touch with that this last few days. 'It's needing to get away. I needed to get away last time.'

'Mhmm. Needed to get away.' Michael paused and waited to see where Peter would take it.

Peter frowned and shook his head. 'But it was different. A different getting away.'

Michael empathised with Peter's facial expression, returning the frown, but again with a hint of questioning curiosity. 'Different? A different kind of getting away?'

Peter nodded, but said nothing. They remained in silence for a short while. Peter spoke first. 'Getting away is a real theme at the moment and yet, it feels so deep, like it goes back a long way.'

'Like it's been around for you for a long while.'

Again Peter nodded, but with less head movement this time, and again a silence followed. Michael felt his senses keying up. The silences had become suddenly more intense, really silent. A stillness that seemed almost otherworldly seemed to have become present in the room.

Such intense experiences can become present where clients are engaging with material at depth, and where the counsellor is holding contact with the client. Sensory distortion can be unsettling for the therapist; however, it is vital that they stay with the client and be ready to journey with them wherever they need to go. These events in therapy do not occur with all clients, but when they do, there is likely to be something highly significant emerging into the client's awareness.

Peter went to speak, but closed his mouth, tightening his lips and releasing the air through his nose as he did so. He sat in silence for a moment or two. He knew he was having difficulty making sense of it. Getting away, got to get away. Got to get away. What was he getting away from? The counselling – sure. Michael – maybe. From his mother – yes. From …? He sat thinking. But his thoughts were melting as other sensations came to the fore.

Michael sat waiting, holding as best he could feelings of warmth for Peter, wanting to hold him in his process, holding his sense of trust in that process, in that wonderful actualising tendency that he knew would push whatever needed to emerge into the light of Peter's awareness. He loved the process. Loved the sense of growth, change, movement, realised potential. It was why he was a counsellor. He loved that sense of making a difference, of being part of that process of growth. And he knew that it helped him grow too. Yet it was more than that. He put his thought on hold as Peter was starting to speak again.

'Getting away.' Peter's face had changed and he looked suddenly small, like he was retreating into the chair, and the chair was retreating into the wall. Michael felt his own goosebumps. He'd been here before with clients. He knew something important was happening. Something deep, and this was a moment where he just had to be fully present, had to get it right. His eyes were suddenly watery. He held his focus on Peter.

'Got to go away.' The voice didn't sound like Peter's and yet it was. But it sounded so childlike.

Michael adjusted to the reality of the moment. He was probably sitting with a
child, at least, a childlike part of Peter. He spoke softly, simply. 'Peter's got to
go away.'

Peter was looking down. He suddenly looked up. His eyes were wide and round,
not his usual expression at all. More goosebumps.

'It's OK.' Michael smiled. 'It's OK, Peter.'

Peter was hearing himself speak and speaking at the same time. He'd never felt
like this. He was stuck, captivated – no, wrong word, mesmerised by what
was happening. He was himself and yet he wasn't, but he was. Everything
seemed different, bigger somehow. He felt small, very small. It felt weird and
yet it felt familiar too, like it was a place he knew. As he sat and looked towards
Michael he ... now it was weird, and yet it still wasn't. It was like a movie on
the wall, like he was seeing something replaying. He felt his skin pricking in his
back, his arms, his legs. He sat, staring just to the left of where Michael was
sitting. He saw Michael and yet he was compelled to watch the images that
were there, on the wall, and they weren't really on the wall. And as he watched
he could feel, and the feelings were connected to what he was seeing.

Michael stayed calm, not moving, not wanting to in any way disturb what was
happening for Peter. He felt extremely alert. This was going to be a crucial
moment in the counselling process, a moment of movement, as he recalled
Rogers referring to critical points within the therapeutic process. Moments of
shift, change, when something emerged, happened, connected. He stayed holding his complete focus on Peter, an attitude of loving expectation.

Peter could feel anxiety as he watched himself in the dark, no, not watched himself, he wasn't seeing himself, but he was seeing though his own eyes, but they
were low, he was low. The door handle was high, he was reaching up to it.
He was thirsty, his throat was dry, so dry, and he was miserable, sleepy. He was
cold as well, he wanted to be warm, he wanted someone to ... he wanted, he
just wanted.

He could feel the warm air of the room touch his face as the door opened, it was dark
and he could hear strange noises ahead of him. Muffled, couldn't understand
them. He couldn't turn on the light, he didn't know where the switch was – felt
he might not have been able to reach it. He heard his voice. He wasn't speaking,
but he heard his voice. 'Mummy. Mummy. Can I have a drink of water?'

The noises stopped, abruptly. He heard movement. The light came on, the bedside
light. He saw his mother, his mummy, he wasn't sure which she was – his
mummy, but ... Peter was flooded with feeling and emotions. He was suddenly
two people. He could feel utter confusion and shock – coming from himself,
from somewhere deep, from within his smallness – and absolute horror from
himself as he was looking on. He was transfixed, staring at the image before
him, but was it before him, was it in his head? He couldn't think about it, he
just sat, standing, watching, frozen, horrified. Who was that man? Who was
he? He didn't know him. It wasn't his daddy, his father.

'Go away. Go a-waaaay!' The voice screeched in his brain, but it wasn't in his
head but outside of his head as well. His mummy, his mother, screaming at
him to go away. But he couldn't go. He couldn't move. Peter the adult sat,

unable to move. Peter the child stood, unable to move. Both icy cold. Both connected in time in the horror of a singular moment of experience.

'Will you go back to your room, NOW!'

It felt like an eternity as the scene continued to be played out. He wasn't moving, either then or now. Suddenly, abruptly, the scene moved, he must have been turning and running in the dark back to his room. Running into darkness. All he could see was darkness. All he could feel was darkness, it swirled around him, then, now, time, space, everything, everywhere. He closed his eyes and felt his body jerk. He was back in the present. This present. There weren't two presents, but there had been, there was, there is. Where was he? He was disorientated in space, in time, in consciousness.

Michael saw the jerk and the confused look. 'It's OK, Peter, it's OK. I'm here. You're safe. You've had a really bad . . .' Michael realised he didn't know what to say. 'Something you've seen, remembered. It's OK. Take your time.' He sought to reassure him. He took the assumption that he had experienced something awful – given the expression on his face – and something from a long time ago again given the special distortion. Peter was looking directly at him, right into his eyes, his own wide open in disbelief.

'I . . .'

'Take your time, Peter, no rush, take your time.' He didn't say 'it's OK', he'd said it once to reassure Peter, not sure whether he was talking to the small Peter or the adult one, but Peter was back in adult – at least he thought so, and it plainly wasn't OK.

An interesting point. 'It's OK' can be used to reassure, but when it is used in a context where what the client is experiencing or conveying is not OK, it is likely to be therapeutically unhelpful. Sometimes it might be more valuable to say 'you're OK' to reassure.

Peter opened his mouth, and closed it again. He again shook his head. He felt numb, his arms, legs felt heavy. His breathing was shallow though he wasn't aware of it. What he had seen, what he had experienced was somehow deeply familiar yet forgotten. It wasn't something on the wall, something from outside of his experience. He knew, *he knew*, that what he had seen and experienced had happened and in a sense was happening to him again. He had seen his mother, he had heard her, he had seen the man – and he had no idea who he was – and he had felt frozen, unable to move, and then the swirling darkness. He still felt frozen but it wasn't a cold frozen now, a numb frozen better described it. He closed his eyes as a sudden surge of emotion swept into his body and into his eyes. And somewhere in among the swirl of everything in his head, his heart, the pit of his stomach, he found himself thinking a crazy thought, a stupid, insignificant thought. Of all the things to come to mind – he never got his glass of water.

In that moment of thinking he looked over to the table – it had a glass of water on it. He somewhat shakily reached over and picked it up, and took a sip. He hesitated, then took another, and another. He continued, gulping down the whole glass. He somehow needed to drink it, had to drink it, it was more than a glass of water. He was compelled to finish it. It was somehow satisfying, and yet not satisfying enough. But in that moment he felt some of the numbness passing, he felt himself coming back into himself – if that was the right way to describe it, and he wasn't at all sure that it was.

He took a deep breath, 'Oohhh,' and blew the air out. 'I just experienced something from my childhood that I had forgotten. It's a shock.'

Michael didn't smile, but nodded ever so slightly. 'Yes, I can see the shock in your face. Something from childhood.'

While Michael has empathised with the shock, he has left Peter with a focus on the fact of his having experienced something from childhood. Good use of empathy, conveying that the shock has been noted, but the underlying cause remains the primary focus.

'It was like I relived it but watched it. It's weird, I feel really strange. But it's like it's something I'd forgotten but now remember, like I had forgotten I knew it but now it's real, vivid.' He described what he had experienced. Michael listened, saying little, responding minimally as Peter described what was occurring.

'When the light came on in the bedroom, I . . . I just froze, I was . . . I don't know. I don't know.' He felt emotions rising once more, shock, horror, confusion, and feeling utterly alone in himself with what had happened, and what had come back into his conscious awareness. Peter put his head in his hands, his eyes were screwed up tight. He didn't know what to say, he-just-didn't-know. He sat, head in hands for a short while, feeling waves of confusion inside himself, disorientated, just not knowing what to say or do.

'You don't know – like Peter in the bedroom you don't know, frozen, just don't know . . .' Michael sought to empathise, speaking softly, not wishing to disturb the processing taking place with Peter.

'I saw their faces – my mother and this man – he had really dark hair, a moustache, he looked startled, he was staring at me like he didn't know what to do. I saw his eyes – dark, wide-eyed, they seemed – they seem – wild looking. I can see them now.' He paused before continuing. 'I can see them now.'

'Those dark, wild eyes, yes, so clear, so clear.'

Peter had closed his eyes again, feeling the raw emotion in his heart, his chest was tight, his throat was dry. 'I need some water.' He froze as he said it, and looked up at Michael.

Michael nodded. There was nothing he needed to say. Peter was making a connection and he needed the freedom and space to do it. Michael didn't need to add anything. Peter was nodding as well, and taking a deep breath. Peter reached over to the jug, filled the glass and drank deeply from it once again.

Peter continued with what he had experienced. 'My mother started shouting at me, telling me to "go away!". I can hear her voice so clearly. And I remember not knowing what to do, and just standing there, and then I turned and ran into the dark, back to my room. I don't remember anything after that, just running back into the darkness. I guess I must have gone back to bed, I guess, I don't know, I just don't know.' He looked at Michael. 'It did really happen, didn't it, I mean, it's not my imagination, is it?'

'Does it feel like imagination, Peter?' Michael did not want to confirm the experience just at the moment, he wanted Peter to assess it for himself, although he knew that this kind of really vivid remembering was, in his experience, highly likely to be true.

Peter was shaking his head. 'No. I know it happened, it's just such a shock to suddenly remember it, and to see it, so vividly, I mean, I was there . . . part of me still feels there, so real, so . . .' He couldn't find the words.

'Mhmm, part of you still there, still in the experience, in the reality and the vividness of it.'

Peter took a deep breath and closed his eyes again. He felt suddenly very shaky, like his body was reacting. He could feel himself trembling. Michael had noticed it.

Sometimes a physical reaction to this kind of vivid re-experiencing takes place within the session. If it does not, the counsellor would be advised to point out to the client that they might experience some kind of reaction. This can obviously be important if a client is travelling home alone, or driving. It is good practice to be able to offer clients time and space after sessions to compose themselves before leaving.

'Shock's really into your body, Peter, just take it calmly, steadily, don't push yourself.' He guessed that maybe he was experiencing some kind of after-shock, or maybe this was a psychosomatic reaction to what had emerged into Peter's awareness. Either way, he wanted to be sure that Peter was OK, and to keep reassuring him. Clearly, the whole event that had been remembered was one that Peter – whatever part of himself was present – needed reassurance about. He wasn't sure how the event was later handled, what message Peter got from it about himself and how he internalised it. But he knew that it wasn't going to be very healthy, and was clearly psychologically damaging to a child who had simply wanted a glass of water.

Peter could feel himself trembling, his teeth were chattering, he felt strangely cold and numb, light-headed. He gritted his teeth and closed his eyes again, seeking to regain some control of his body.

Michael felt a huge urge to hold Peter, to offer him physical reassurance as clearly what had happened was now affecting him at a very physical level. He got up and moved over to Peter, kneeling down beside him. Peter instinctively leaned his head towards him and Michael put his arms around him, holding him steadily.

How do you make the judgement as to when it is appropriate to move over to a client and, as in this case, initiate physical contact? The person-centred counsellor will seek to be sufficiently self-aware to know where the motivation is coming from although, as can happen, it can be an utter spontaneous urge that simply feels right. Perhaps the best litmus test is 'when in doubt, don't', but always check in supervision in case there is something within the counsellor that is stopping them from responding through physical contact when it is appropriate and has therapeutic value.

Immediately another rush of emotion tore through Peter. He held Michael back, well, clung to him would be more accurate. Michael felt the strength of his grip. He continued with his own hold, feeling the pressure on his body but knowing that this was such a crucial moment in the therapeutic process. Had Peter ever been held quite like this – by his mother or father, by another man, by anyone – as a child or as an adult? The power of Peter's grip was uncomfortable but Michael was determined not to break the connection. So he stayed, holding him. Neither of them spoke. The empathic connection, the communication of unconditional warmth and acceptance, the genuineness of the moment did not need words. It was beyond words. Two men, one in deep pain and shock, one staying open to his own reactions to what had occurred, both holding each other in a moment of human solidarity in the face of traumatic experience.

Michael felt Peter take a deep breath, and felt his grip relax a little. 'Thanks.' He pulled back slightly, and Michael mirrored him by relaxing his grip and also relaxing back.

'I needed to reach out, Peter, I hope it helped.'

Peter nodded. 'Never held anyone like that before – or been held. Feel odd about it now.' He pulled back a little more and let go of Michael. As Peter sat back in his chair Michael asked if he wanted him to stay where he was.

In the moment it was right, but then, after the moment has passed, another aspect of Peter cuts in that is uncomfortable about the physical contact. He's done something new. It felt good, but probably conditioning is telling him that it was an odd thing to have happened. And yet it felt good. There is an inner conflict which may be expressed, or may be set aside by the client who does not want to engage with it, seeking to preserve one or other of the two reactions.

'No. I'm OK. Thanks.'

Michael returned to his chair.

Peter felt he needed to say something. 'I don't think I've ever been held, or held, like that.'

'New experience, holding and being held?'

Peter nodded. 'It felt, well, not sure what I was feeling, I just needed that. Thanks. Feels odd now, though.'

'Mhmm.'

'Yes, but no, it . . .' Peter didn't know what to say. He had held people, but not like that. He thought of Melanie, and of girlfriends he'd had in the past. But somehow this had been different, so intense. The fleeting thought went through his mind about whether he was gay, but he knew he wasn't. Peter shook his head. He closed his eyes. 'I needed that, needed something, someone. There wasn't anyone when it happened. I don't think I talked about it to anyone. And that man – never remember seeing him again. Really don't know what happened, but I don't remember him again.'

'No one to hold you, no one to talk to, and . . .'

Michael didn't finish; Peter was shaking his head. '. . . don't ever remember being held or hugged or anything like that.' He felt a sense of aloneness as he spoke. 'It must have affected me, Michael, must have been bad for me.'

Michael nodded. 'Yes, you really wonder what effect it had on you, how bad it must have been.'

Peter was feeling quite quiet, his thoughts had been racing, his head spinning, but he now felt like he was looking at something sort of separated off from himself although it felt close and part of him at the same time, at least he knew it was. It was strange, almost otherworldly. Nothing seemed somehow solid or safe – at least, the feeling struck him that that was how it was. He felt disturbed, uncomfortable, unsure and uncertain. At least the shaking had stopped, but his head felt very strange.

'She was having an affair and no one knew – I guess – but me. And since then she's hated me for it.' Peter hadn't planned to say the last sentence, but he did and he heard himself saying it and he knew that, yes, that was precisely how it was, how it had been. He knew, she hated him. They shared a secret except that he'd forgotten about it, lost his memory of it. 'So, what do I do now?' Peter had glanced at the clock. Time was passing and there were only about 10 minutes or so left of the session.

'What do you want to do, Peter?'

'I don't know. I need time to let this sink in.' He shook his head. 'It just seems to make sense of things, I mean, why she is as she is with me, and has been all these years. I know I have to say something to her, but not now, not yet, it's all too close.'

'Mhmm. That sounds very reasonable, Peter. Take your time. It's a huge shock. Yes, it may well help you to make sense of a lot of the things that have happened to you. And, yes, you don't think the time is right to say anything.' Michael really wanted to communicate his trust in Peter to make the choices that he needed to make.

'I never expected anything like this.' Peter looked up to the ceiling as he spoke. He didn't know why, maybe he was looking to God, to some unseen influence to help him to come to terms with what had just occurred – and what had occurred so many years ago.

'No.' Michael paused. 'No,' he quietly repeated, 'how could you?'

'I couldn't. I didn't know. It's horrible but I'm glad I do know now. I'm glad I've remembered, Michael, and I'm sure that this evening is going to be a turning point in my life.'

Michael nodded. 'That's how you'd like to see it, how you'd like it to be, a turning point in your life.'

'It has to be . . . it has to be.'

'Yeah.' Michael found himself taking a deep breath and smiling across to Peter although with a still serious expression.

'And I'm wondering what did happen next, I mean, why did that guy never . . .' Peter was shaking his head. 'Why did he never appear again – or did he and I've forgotten that too?'

'Mhmm, why didn't he appear again, or, as you say, did he and you can't remember.'

'I don't think he did. I really don't. I've got a kind of hunch that maybe, well, maybe he kind of left the scene. And maybe it was a one night stand, maybe. Where my father was, well, I've no idea. It was madness – three children in the house and she has a man back with her. Christ, the risk.' He shook his head. 'She must have really wanted him.'

'Big risk, and, well, we know what happened, and yes, maybe what you say is true.' Michael did not want to get into speculation.

Peter went quiet again. He was feeling a bit more like himself. He knew he had to head off soon and needed to get his head into gear once more. It had been an hour of his life that he didn't expect he'd ever forget.

'Thanks for today, I really mean that. It wasn't easy – it was horrible – but thanks. I needed it. I need time now to really make sense of it all and decide what to do next. I'll be back next week – no more missed sessions.' He wondered whether at some level or whatever he kind of knew what was happening inside himself; maybe he'd avoided last week to avoid what he was experiencing this week. He didn't know. But it did leave him wondering. However, he was sure that he needed to continue with the counselling. He really had to make sense of all of this and, well, maybe take a fresh stock of his life, his options, but with the added awareness of what had happened in the past, how it might have affected him, and his relationship with his mother. He heard Michael respond but he didn't really take it in.

'A lot to think about, and I look forward to sharing this process with you and I hope helping you to get to where you need to be in yourself and in your life.'

'Thanks. I hope I get there. I'll see you next week.'

The session closed and Michael left, and while he had calmed down he was aware that his thought process had picked up again. Yes, he thought, I have a lot to think about. And I also need to talk about it too – he was thinking about Melanie, and thinking about giving her a call that evening to talk about the counselling session.

Michael returned to the counselling room after seeing Peter out. He was exhausted. He'd put the kettle on as he had passed the kitchen – he knew he needed something before he felt ready to see his next client. Such a powerful session, so intense, and such implications for Peter and how he has been virtually throughout his life. He often thought of life like a kaleidoscope that gets turned and, without doubt, Peter's psychological kaleidoscope had just been turned – and very abruptly. He paused. That word again, abruptly. He wasn't surprised, it seemed to capture a theme and he wondered how many other times things had occurred in Peter's life in an abrupt manner, and how, if that was the case, Peter had developed in response.

He went out to the kitchen, poured his tea and returned to write his notes of the session.

Points for discussion

- How did you react to Peter reliving his past experience? Has it changed your view of Peter, his mother, and how might it impact on you as a therapist working with Peter?
- How would you explore this in supervision? What would be the key areas that you would want to bring?
- What do you feel enabled Peter to reconnect with his memory? How did Michael contribute to this?
- What issues came to mind concerning the physical contact in the session given that Michael is gay?
- What other elements of the session do you feel are significant?
- Write notes for the counselling session.

Supervision session 2

14 October

Michael had begun by describing what had been happening in his sessions with Peter. Suzy listened and noted a sense that Michael was uneasy. She couldn't quite put her finger on it, but there was something about the way he spoke that left her feeling that in some way he was not comfortable with what was happening. She noted it and waited to see if it would pass.

'So, he has reconnected with a memory from his early childhood and now he has to somehow integrate that into himself, and into his life and his relationships, particularly towards his mother.' Michael paused. 'You know, I really feel for him. It's hard to imagine quite what it must be like to recover a memory like that. I mean, I guess at some level, he knew. I mean, the memory was stored somewhere, but out of reach – at least from his waking consciousness, if I can put it like that.'

Suzy empathised with his feeling. 'Yes, something about his situation really touches you.'

Michael nodded. He'd been left with a clear image of the look on Peter's face as he had relived that experience. It had made a profound impression. So much expression. Michael felt quiet and he simply nodded in response to Suzy.

Suzy noted the silence and it felt different, meaningful in some way. It felt important to stay therapeutically connected with Michael. She wasn't his therapist
and she had no intention of drifting into that place, yet she sensed that something was happening for Michael and she knew she needed to help him. Nothing
outwardly, nothing he had particularly said, but it was a sense she had – call it
an intuition perhaps – and she had learned to trust such subtle promptings.

Michael looked across at Suzy. She seemed very calm, a slight smile but without
smiling, seemingly inviting him to say more, to express what was present for
him. He took a deep breath though his lips remained tight. After a few more
moments he began to share his feelings.

'I somehow seem to be feeling quite overwhelmed by the magnitude of what Peter
is facing. Here we are, talking about it, and somewhere out there Peter is doing
whatever he needs to do to come to terms with what has happened.'

'Mhmm, somewhere out there. And it affects you.' Suzy kept her response minimal, and open. She waited.

'It does affect me. I mean, I know I trust his process, and all that. I know that the
actualising tendency will seek a constructive expression in response to what
has occurred. I know that . . .' His voice seemed to trail off.

'You know that . . .' Suzy reflected his words and his style of speaking.

Michael was shaking his head, yes he did know it, and yet . . . Somehow, and he
was somewhat surprised and unnerved by it, but he could feel a sense of
unease, of somehow not being quite so sure. 'I do know that, and yet . . .'

'And yet . . .?'

Michael was shaking his head again. 'It seems so immense.'

'Mhmm. Such an immense thing to face.'

Michael was aware that he felt quiet inside as he was speaking. Yes, he knew the
actualising tendency moved people towards fuller functioning, towards a more
fulfilling way of being, or at least a way of being that most effectively met the
individual's perceived needs. And yet . . . There was something about what
Peter was facing up to, and it seemed to be touching something very deep
within Michael as he sat there, reflecting on the therapeutic process.

Michael closed his eyes. 'Where do you begin, I mean, where does Peter begin? His
world can never be the same. He knows something, really knows something,
about his mother, about himself. He knows that his mother rejected him, refused
to meet his needs, and in a highly emotional moment when, as a young child, he
sees this strange man in bed with her. I mean, what did he think? Well, maybe
he didn't, maybe he just felt but was unable to process the feelings.' Michael
paused and thought back to the last session. 'Well, he's re-engaged with them
to some degree. What it will lead to, how he will become, I don't know.'

Suzy responded to what she felt was present. 'Sounds like you want to know.'

'Yes, I really wish I could see how this is going to turn out. One moment in that
session he seemed determined to leave – oh yes, he talked about wanting to
leave like a bat out of hell – reference to some record – I don't know, not my
scene. But he really seemed to have connected with that and then . . .' Michael
was speaking more slowly as he made a connection. 'Must have felt like hell in
that bedroom, must have not known what to do, or what he wanted to do. Run?

But which way?' He shook his head. 'Poor kid. Didn't deserve that, and, well, maybe the rejection started then, or maybe it had already begun. Kind of feel the latter otherwise you'd think that his mother would have been more caring towards him. But he doesn't remember that. Of course, he could be screening that out in order to maintain his primary sense as a not-good-enough boy, as someone only deserving of rejection.' Michael paused again. 'Guess it gets to me.'

Suzy nodded, and she felt it was important to help Michael clarify what he was experiencing. Peter was affecting him and that was OK, it was a sign of relationship between them, but she also needed to be sure that Michael was able to hear Peter, to hear what Peter wanted to communicate and for it not to get lost among Michael's own reactions.

'Gets to you, what he went through, how it affected him, how he is now.' Suzy sought to not only empathise with what had just been said, but draw together the threads that she was experiencing Michael communicating to her.

Michael had closed his eyes again and was aware of a sense of his own identity as a man, what that meant to him. He wasn't sure how his thoughts had wandered to this theme, but that was how it was. 'Leaves me thinking of myself and what it means for me to be a man, Suzy.'

'Mhmm, wondering what that does mean for you, and for Peter.'

'I'm not like him, not been in that place, can't really identify with it and yet there is something about what he has told me that sort of resonates, but I can't put a memory or an experience to it.' Michael was frowning as he struggled to make sense of his experience.

'Like there's something about you that resonates with Peter?'

Michael was shaking his head. 'No, not exactly. I'm not sure. It's not an experiential thing in the sense of feeling I've had his experience. I don't have a sense of rejection, I really don't and I've not unearthed anything in my own therapy, so I feel OK about that. And yet, there's still something that really touches me.' As he spoke he felt an upwelling of emotion. He found himself taking a deep breath and feeling suddenly fired up, angry. He wasn't sure where that had come from, but it was present for him as he looked over towards Suzy who continued to sit quietly yet with a sense of curious interest in her expression.

'Mhmm, that something, that something . . .' Suzy did not want to direct Michael towards any conclusion, or to actually help him to resolve his experience. Rather she wanted to give him time to reach his own conclusion which could involve him being given the space to connect with an aspect of himself, or something within his own experience that had relevance to the relationship he was forming with Peter.

He listened to Suzy, to the way she spoke, lowly and quietly. Yes, he thought, that something. And he could feel a bit of fire now, 'bloody woman', he heard himself say with some degree of passion. Suzy was slightly taken aback by the abruptness. She guessed her body language must have communicated this. She voiced her feeling, seeking to maintain her own transparency in the supervisory relationship. 'Where did that come from?' The moment she said it she realised she hadn't empathised but had rather been unable to stop herself from conveying surprise.

Michael shrugged, he didn't know and he didn't care much. 'I don't know. She pisses me off. Peter's a nice guy, but he didn't deserve any of this.'

'You really like him.'

'I do.' Another pause. 'I'd hate to have to face up to what he is going through. I mean, how does it affect you? I know, you know, theoretically, and I've seen and experienced how crap in childhood affects people, gets to them, messes them up. But Peter's not messed up – he's got a good job, but he's stuck at home, wanting to get away and yet desperate to feel his mother's love – and she's not giving it.' A thought struck him and he was voicing it as he was thinking it. 'Surely a boy has a right to love from his mother.'

'A right to be loved.'

'Well, yes, I was loved.'

'Mhmm, you were loved so Peter should have been loved.'

'Yes. Dammit, I know it isn't that way for many people, and I know that love is often quite conditional – you know, I'll only love you if ... but ...' Michael paused, he knew what he was about to say, but suddenly the words weren't right. He'd wanted to say that conditional love was better than no love, but he wasn't sure. Suddenly he wasn't sure. It was an idea that he'd been aware of but it was suddenly very present for him. He didn't know why – why in this particular moment it seemed to have deeper significance – but he knew the thought wasn't something he could put into words and own.

Suzy noted the hesitation and responded, '... but ...?'

'Caught myself, wanted to say conditional love is better than no love, and yet, well, I guess I just don't know.' He grimaced. 'Love, so much comes back to it – what is it? Why the hell is it so important? But it is. We need it, like oxygen, the child crying for attention I guess in the moment that someone responds feels different, is somehow reassured, able to feel in some way that he or she is deserving of attention. It's so difficult. So much goes on before we even have the words to describe it. How can we really understand what the child actually experiences? It must be so isolated, suddenly alone in the world having had nine months in the womb – warm, nourished, floating.' Michael was aware that he was talking a lot but he also knew it was something he felt passionate about. Somewhere deep inside himself, within his own memory lay the experience of his own time in the womb, his own birth and sudden entrance into a world no longer warm and protective, a world in which you now had to attract attention to get needs met. He knew he must carry this memory at some level, that we all did.

'Huge contrast, and the sense of isolation strikes you.'

Michael was nodding. 'Yes, I mean, suddenly you're on your own and yet, have you really got a sense of self? I mean, at what age does the child really begin to be able to own the sense of separation. It happens the moment the umbilical cord is cut – and I often wonder whether that occurs too soon, whether it should be left intact during those first – I don't know how long – minutes held by the mother.' Michael paused again. 'Oh, I don't know, there's no doubt some good medical reason, but I just wonder if it might somehow ease the transition in some way.'

Suzy was very struck by the idea but did not know whether there were medical grounds for cutting the cord sooner rather than later.

Michael continued, bringing his thoughts back to Peter. 'I mean, was he wanted from the start? Or was he only rejected at the time of the incident when he was a child, and it continued from then?' Michael shook his head. 'I really hope he felt love when he was born.' There were tears in Michael's eyes; it had really got to him. Something about the idea of being born, of the isolation, and maybe of not experiencing that mysterious something called love. His heart went out to Peter, and he suddenly felt anger towards his mother.

Suzy noticed the expression change on Peter's face – from sadness to a really heavy frown and a suddenly tightened jaw. 'The sadness looks like it has been replaced by anger?'

'Mhmm?' Michael looked up; he had been in his own thoughts – well, in truth, in his own feelings. 'Yeah, well, just thinking of his mother.' He took a deep breath.

'You feel anger towards her?' Suzy was aware that she wasn't empathising with what Michael was saying, but tending more towards speculating, and yet she was also saying nothing that hadn't been conveyed by Michael through the combination of his words and facial expression.

'Yes, I do.' He tightened his lips once more as he thought about what he was thinking and feeling. 'I have to be honest with myself, these feelings are there, and, well, I guess they may get in the way.'

'In the way?' Suzy was inviting Michael to say more about his experience.

'Of my being open, well, maybe more transparent, towards Peter.'

'So your feelings towards his mother stop you being transparent?'

'Well, I mean, they are feelings that if I was to be transparent I'd have to express.'

'Mhmm.' Suzy didn't say any more, allowing what Michael had said to stay with him. She sat and waited. Her thoughts were along the lines of, 'so you feel these things, why hide them away?'

'I guess for me it is a question of whether I should be venting anger here and therefore being free of it when I am with Peter, or should I simply understand my anger from my process here and be open to the possibility of revealing it to Peter?'

Suzy found herself nodding. She felt that Michael had really summed up the dilemma well, and yet she was also aware of her own instinctive reaction, which she voiced. 'Why not both, vent it, understand it and be open to expressing it with Peter?'

'I don't want to collude with his view.'

'You don't want to collude with his view of his mother?'

'Yes.' Michael knew that this wasn't right. 'But I wouldn't be colluding, I mean, I'd be owning my stuff, wouldn't I?'

'You would. So long as you say it in a way that conveys it.'

Michael nodded. 'Yes, I can't start saying stuff about her, but maybe I can be open to what I feel.' He frowned. 'And I know that, I know that I have to be open to my feelings, and yet there is something about this situation that is leaving me reluctant or unsure. And I need to understand why.'

'Unsure about being transparent, something about your relationship with Peter, or his relationship with his mother, or . . .' She didn't get a chance to continue; Michael continued for her.

'. . . or more likely my relationship with myself.'

'Mhmm, something about your relationship to yourself.' Suzy was puzzled, unsure quite what Michael was getting at. She must have conveyed that in her own facial expression.

'You look puzzled.'

'I am. I'm not sure what you mean by relationship with yourself in a person-centred context, and I don't want to now go and direct us into a theoretical discussion, rather stay with what it is that you experience when you say "relationship with yourself".'

Michael paused but only briefly. 'It's like how I react to my own reactions. It's like I feel what I feel for Peter, for his mother. They are present within me and yet, well, they're not me. I mean, it's like the feelings are present and I am experiencing them, but I am somehow not them.'

'So you're not your feelings, but you have feelings?'

'That's right, and there is something about Peter and his mother – and you know, I realise I don't know her name, and part of me is curious and another part of me doesn't want to know! But there is something about . . .' Michael looked down as he thought about what it was he was trying to say. It seemed difficult to put into words, and yet important. He was aware of anxiety within himself. 'It's making me feel anxious, I'm not sure why.'

'Mhmm, something about that relationship and it leaves you feeling anxious . . .'

Michael couldn't grasp what it was that was present for him. It seemed like it was out of reach, on the edge of his awareness in some way. Present and yet somehow – he was going to think distant, but it wasn't distant. It was close, and he was struck by the sense that maybe it was too close. 'There's a something and I can't get hold of it, but I sense that it is getting hold of me.'

'So something, linked to their relationship, leaving you anxious, hard to get hold of and yet it has in some way got hold of you.' Suzy was really trying to get hold of what Michael was experiencing and communicating. It wasn't simply a reflection she had offered, she was experiencing greater depth than the simple mirroring of Michael's words. To her they were both on a journey, feeling their way forward towards . . .? She sat, seeking to remain open to what was present within her as she also maintained her focus on Michael and what he was trying to connect with.

Michael sat, tight-lipped again. He couldn't find it, connect with it. He was shaking his head. He opened up his hands almost as though he as trying to physically get hold of something, but he couldn't. He had tensed them along with his fingers, as though he was holding some large invisible ball in front of his chest. 'I can't get hold of it.'

A thought struck Suzy and she felt a strong urge to say something that wasn't directly linked to what Michael was saying, and yet . . . She trusted this instinct. 'Pre-verbal?'

Michael nodded. 'Maybe. If so, then, it may mean something happened earlier that affected Peter and it's locked up in his pre-verbal experiencing and it's leaving it so difficult for us to get hold of it with our adult, word-based thinking and feeling.'

They both sat for a while in silence, each contemplating what had been said, and the implication. Of course, neither knew the reality, in many respects it was speculation, and yet . . . Suzy had felt a strong sense of the idea that the struggle was to put something into words that was perhaps contained within Peter's experience in a form that wasn't word-based. And she also believed that everyone had that place in themselves for everyone had a pre-verbal phase of existence where experiences were processed in a very different way.

Michael was aware of feeling rather detached, of sitting as a kind of observer of himself and the dialogue he was having with Suzy. He voiced his experience. 'It's leaving me feeling rather detached – watching myself and our conversation.' He paused to scratch his left shoulder which was itching. He even felt detached from the itch as well. It wasn't a feeling he had when he had arrived earlier, it had rather developed during the session, but more particularly these last 10 minutes or so. And he was aware that the supervision session was nearly over.

'Like you're detached from what's happening?'

'Observing. Like I'm not really feeling.' He snorted. 'What was I saying earlier about not showing my feelings about Peter's mother? Now I don't seem to be in touch with feelings at all!'

Suzy responded, 'Like you're cut off from feelings. They're there but you're not experiencing them, or they're just not there?'

'I'm sure they're there but I'm back from them in some way. Funny, I'm still thinking back to what we discussed earlier. Not showing feelings then, and now can't.'

'I'm wondering what was the process we went through – you went through – to reach this place and what significance that journey had, what were the main features.'

'Having feelings and not being them. Being uncertain, no, anxious, about transparency. Almost like I approached the idea of being transparent but then, well, here I am being anything but transparent.'

'You're being as you are. We don't understand what is happening, but you are being as you are, as you need to be, and it seems to me you are bringing it into our relationship and communicating it. It's just so very difficult to communicate and there is this sense of being detached within yourself, if that is the right way of expressing it. And there is the pre-verbal idea we touched into as well. It's all very powerful stuff. And I sense you as being present, but in the midst of, I don't know, a . . . a . . . , well, a something.'

'Yes, it's like a something that I can't put into words. There's something about Peter not being able to connect with something. That word keeps coming up now. But that's how it is. He's connected to an experience in childhood – a really painful and difficult and wholly rejecting experience. He wouldn't have been able to make rational sense of it, but maybe blamed himself in some way.

That's speculation. But anyway. And maybe behind it all is something else. And that's also speculation.'

'Yes, lot of speculation all of a sudden. We don't know. We really don't know, and perhaps we have to accept that and be open to that not knowing. It's OK not to know.'

A broad grin broke out on Michael's face, and he could suddenly feel some kind of change taking place inside of himself. It was clearing, he was feeling clearer. It was like a fog had lifted. Yes, he thought, yes. He was smiling even more as Suzy asked him what had happened.

'Maybe for us, but for Peter, he's got to know something, he's got to know that he's loved. He's got to feel that love. He's got to have that affirmation that in the eyes of his mother he is lovable. Back to needing love like oxygen. He knows he needs it, but that need, that urge is being driven from his pre-verbal development.' Michael was feeling clearer still as he developed his train of thought and continued to speak. 'He's got to know. He can't allow himself to doubt it. He's got to know. He's got to feel love – and I imagine as well there is a part of him in utter fear of opening himself to the possibility for fear of rejection once again.' He felt the goosebumps breaking out on his back and neck, and somehow for Michael there was a very clear knowing that what he was saying did reflect Peter's experience. And he felt so different, so much lighter.

'You look more alert, more present somehow, more sort of animated,' Suzy had been struck by a change, 'and it feels like there's more connection as well.'

Michael nodded. 'I feel lighter. Something's cleared, shifted. It seems like I needed time wallowing in it before I could emerge from it.'

'I'm aware that we don't have much time left, but I want to say that it may have needed time. Perhaps the experience you have had represents something happening for you that is either about processing your reaction to Peter and his mother, or it is something that may leave you relating to him from a different place within yourself. Maybe?'

Michael took a deep breath, and then paused. He cocked his head slightly to one side as he looked over to Suzy. 'You know, it's like I have cleared something but I couldn't tell you for the life of me what it was. But something has happened. Something has changed. It's like ... it's the pre-verbal again. I can't put into words, but there's a shift and there is clarity and lightness. Maybe I'd simply picked up on stuff that I needed to put down, let go of, process – what do we mean by these words?'

'Maybe you have needed to be as you have been this session and, well, we do not know the reason and we do not know the result. We must trust that what has happened has value, even if we cannot explain it.'

The session closed with Michael feeling a strong sense of motivation towards his work with Peter, and yet he noted, as he thought about it on his way home, it wasn't that he wanted to make Peter different or do something. He realised he had been holding those thoughts and feelings, but now he somehow felt himself more accepting. Not a specific acceptance of one thing or another, but a general acceptance of Peter, his mother, the process they were experiencing, and the fact that he was being brought into relationship with that process. Yes, more of a motivation to be in the process. He wondered what would happen next, whether he might be different when he next saw Peter. He didn't know and, in many respects, he was aware of thinking that it didn't matter. He'd be how he needed to be, and yes, yes, maybe how he needed to be would turn out to be more transparent. He smiled as he realised he was looking forward to the next session and to being in the process that was therapy.

CHAPTER 6

Counselling session 8: 'Why didn't she love me?', a cathartic release

20 October

Michael had not lost that enthusiasm. He had, on and off, spent a lot of time the last few days pondering his work with Peter, and wondering how it would develop. He felt himself to be particularly present and sharp as Peter came into the counselling room and sat down. Michael noted that he looked tired, and while he momentarily thought about mentioning it, he resisted, sensing rather that whether or not Peter was tired, he may not wish to be directed into that focus at the start of the session. He didn't know what Peter would want to address. He was curious, particularly after the last session and his own supervision. So he began with an open comment communicating his wonder at what Peter wanted to do with the session.

'So, I'm wondering how you wish to use our time today.'

Peter sat quietly for a moment. It had been a dramatic week. He had spent more time with Melanie and was now seriously looking to move out of home, though he was unsure how it would all work out. But he was more convinced than ever of the need to move on. To get away, and yet he also knew he had questions he needed answering, questions that only his mother could answer. The imagery from the previous session had stayed with him. He had felt different and yet he struggled to really describe the difference. It was complex. He seemed very mixed up, and yet he could also get on with his life and put it aside. Thoughts tended to intrude at night. He hadn't been sleeping well.

'Yes, I was thinking about that on the way over. I know I need to continue with the counselling, but it's like I don't really know what to do with it. I'm still coming to terms with the intensity of the last session. Really left me feeling so much.' He paused, aware that he had gone quiet within himself. It had left him with so many mixed up feelings, and yet he also had a sense of clarity as well. He knew he had to move on, more than anything else that was what he had been left with. And yet, somehow that seemed so huge an undertaking while in reality he also felt that it wasn't. 'I need to move on in my life, that's for certain. And being with Melanie is really making me realise how I need to do this – as well as coming here.'

Michael responded, empathising with what Peter had been saying.

Peter continued. 'She has become very important to me, really important. I mean, I'm feeling things about her, towards her, that are so, well, new to me. I mean, I spend a lot of time thinking about her, and we text each other and keep in contact. We talk on the phone on the days that we do not see each other. It really is . . .' He took a slow, deep breath, aware of the sensations in his heart, which felt like it was expanding and wanting to break out of his chest. '. . . it really is quite beautiful.' He smiled, and felt a little embarrassed. But it felt good to have said it; he hadn't told anyone else of how important Melanie was to him. It felt a relief to be saying it here.

Michael was nodding and smiling back. 'She really is important, isn't she?'

Peter nodded. 'I just keep thinking of her, well, most of the time anyway. Then there are times when I drift back into the past and start to wonder what it was all about, and what I really think and feel about mother.' He paused and took another deep breath, shortened this time with a hint of a sigh attached to it as he breathed back out.

'Mmm, feelings and thoughts about your mother.'

That simple response held Peter on his focus and his mother was suddenly more present to him, pushing his feeling for Melanie aside. He didn't like it, he felt angry, irritated. He wanted to think about Melanie, they were lovely thoughts, warm, comforting, reassuring. But his mother, how the hell was he going to move on? He knew he had to but he couldn't see how to, not easily, not without a lot of arguments, and he just didn't want that. He felt too tired.

Empathic responses do not have to be complicated. Simply enabling a client's focus to be held can allow time for other associated feelings to come into awareness. Also, the fact that what was said was quite neutral has meant that there is a genuine space for whatever thoughts and feelings are primary to emerge, without risk of there having been any direction from the counsellor.

Michael waited, wondering whether Peter would focus on his mother, or on Melanie. It seemed to him that there was a real tension suddenly present in the room. Two important women in Peter's life, jostling for supremacy in some way, pulling Peter in two directions.

'But I don't want to talk about her, I mean, I really don't. I kind of want some space from her, and that's sort of why I'm here. I mean, to begin with, yes, get some space, someone to talk to. Now, well, with Melanie in my life, I guess I'm not sure now what to talk about.'

'A real dilemma, which do you talk about, which do you want to bring into the room here?'

Another straightforward but powerful empathic response: not only communicating back what has been said, but also capturing the wider dilemma in the client's life – the tension of having two relationships with two key women, and having to manage that in an effective and satisfying manner.

'I want to bring Melanie in. But I'm not really here to talk about her.' He stopped and pondered for a few moments on a thought that had struck him. 'I guess maybe the time I have with Melanie has sort of replaced some of the time I have here, I mean, I talk to her about things which maybe I had planned to talk about in counselling. And I've talked to her about the past, about what happened in the last session. And that felt so good. She really listened, it really seemed to bring us closer.' He stopped again. He could feel a bit of a lump in his throat. 'She talked about her past as well. She'd had a tough time with her father – real authoritarian. It really touched me. He was so different to my dad who was so much more withdrawn in so many ways. Gave up his power to mother – if he ever had it.' Peter stopped speaking and looked down. He and Melanie had spent one particular evening talking at real depth about her past. He'd spent the evening at her place. The others were out so they had had the place to themselves. It had been a very emotional time and he had stayed the night. They had made love and it had been such a beautiful experience, and he really had felt somehow different. He knew how much he wanted to be with her. Then he remembered his mother's reaction when he had come back the following day, which was Saturday. In fact, he only went back for a change of clothes and then was heading back over to Melanie's to go out into town.

Peter heard Michael respond but he was in his own thoughts. 'My mother completely blanked me because I hadn't come back Friday night.' He was shaking his head. 'When will she accept that I am a man with my own life to lead?'

Michael nodded. 'When will she . . .'

'I mean, for Christ's sake, why can't she let me get on with my life!'

Michael sat, very aware of the tension he could see in Peter's posture. He wanted to allow Peter to be with his feelings, with what was emerging from within him. He knew that his anger and frustration were going to be key factors in whatever choices Peter might make in his situation. He believed that Peter needed to be fully in touch with his own experiencing, and to be able to accurately interpret what became present for him, so that any decisions he took were based on increasing congruence. He also accepted the importance for people of living out in some way their incongruencies, the conditions of worth and the introjects that had contributed to shaping their structure of self until such time as that structure changed.

The structure of self is complex. It is created in order for the person to maintain some continuity of self; however, as the person experiences the therapeutic relationship and begins to re-assess who they are and how they want to be, as they learn to re-define and re-interpret experiences from their past (and present), then the old structure will be forced to change. Of course, certain elements within that self-structure will fight back, seeking to maintain the status quo. However, the new elements, if they are allowed to feel welcome within the therapeutic relationship and outside of the counselling room, and given that they are likely to offer a more satisfying experience for the individual, will want to flourish as well. The client is then caught in what can feel like the middle of a battle-zone. It can be an extremely difficult and confusing time.

'That's what you want, to be allowed to get on with your life.'

Peter felt a reaction to the word 'allowed'. He wanted his own life; he didn't want to feel it was something he had to be allowed to have. 'Dammit, I don't want to be "allowed" a life of my own, I want to take it.' He clenched his teeth. 'I want to take it.' He felt the intensity subside and felt a quietness emerging within himself.

Michael noted that Peter seemed to relax as he finished, or at least his body posture seemed to go from strained to slumped, or something like that. So he recognised that a shift had occurred. It seemed that something else had become present in Peter's experience. He sought to empathise with what was said and the body language. 'You want to take it, and yet . . .'

'And yet I can't. She's my mother. She's a pain, but she's my mum, and I should be there and look after her.'

'She's your mum and you have a real sense that you should be there to look after her, yes?'

Peter was nodding. 'I do, and yet part of me wants to say "no, get on with your life". And I know that's right and yet I also feel this strong urge – no, it isn't so much of an urge, not sure what it is – but I really have this sense that I'd be letting her down, that I should be there.'

'Should be there.' Michael experienced a momentary wonder where the 'should' was coming from.

'Well, yes, you know, after my father died and, well, I mean, it's what sons do, don't they?'

'Do they?'

'Well, yes, I mean, well, I suppose so.' Peter was hesitant. He was feeling confused. He didn't know what to do. 'I mean, I need to be there for her, you know, she wants me around.' He took a deep breath as his thoughts went back to Friday night and, more especially, the reaction he got on the Saturday – and it was still an issue at home.

'You feel you should or need to be around for her. A kind of duty, do you mean, when you say it is what sons do?'

'I suppose so.'

'Well, maybe it isn't exactly like that, maybe it isn't such a sense of duty.' Michael was always concerned when he heard a response like 'I suppose so'; it usually communicated a sense that the client was agreeing with the therapist although not wholeheartedly, so there was a good chance that whatever had been said wasn't strictly accurate. He wanted to afford Peter the opportunity to explore further and engage, if he wanted to, with what was really driving him in his thoughts, feelings and actions towards his mother.

Peter was taking a deep breath. He felt suddenly quite emotional. He heard the words come out of his mouth without having really thought of them. 'Why won't she love me?'

Michael heard the words and they somehow sounded quite childlike in tone. They had been spoken quite quietly and he was aware of the atmosphere suddenly feeling very intense. He suspected a moment of deep connection was occurring, a moment when he needed to be one hundred per cent present in the relationship with Peter.

'Why won't she love Peter.' Michael responded using Peter's name as it simply felt the right response. It was linked to his own sense of the childlike nature of how Peter had spoken.

Peter was taking short, sharp breaths, but otherwise was sitting very still, his hands in his lap, looking suddenly quite small in the chair. Peter could feel the spatial distortion. Peter was going back into some experience; he was connecting with something deeper. Michael knew he had to keep his responses simple and focused, and to hold himself – his awareness and his experiencing – open to what was becoming present.

Peter was shaking his head. He suddenly looked so sad, so incredibly sad. He looked utterly bewildered. 'She doesn't love me.' There was a pause before he continued. 'She hates me.'

'She hates you?'

Peter was nodding. 'Doesn't want me. Never wanted me.'

'Never wanted you?'

'Never wanted me.' Peter's face had changed again, yet subtly, his lower lip was protruding a little more and his face was drawn into a frown. He really looked like a little boy, a sad little boy.

Michael took a risk. He sensed strongly that Peter was talking from the past, that he was very much living out something of his childhood experience, and he knew he needed to match his language to this. He was aware that as an adult Peter had really only spoken of his mother as 'mother', and yet he wouldn't have used that word as a young child. Michael wanted to empathise with Peter as he was present now, and he was in a childlike place within himself. He responded. 'It seems like mummy never wanted Peter.' He deliberately avoided affirming this, hence he said 'it seems like'. Any affirmation of the experience he felt should come from Peter. He didn't want to lodge any interpretations on to what Peter was experiencing.

'No, she didn't want him.' Silence.

Peter was feeling strange, weirdly detached from himself and yet also experiencing himself at the same time. It was like he was experiencing things yet without any real thought or feeling. He wasn't wanted. That was what was present, the simple recognition – a kind of knowing, a deep, deep knowing – that he wasn't wanted. He was kind of numb and yet there was a sadness but he couldn't think of it as sadness; he wasn't thinking with words and concepts. There was simply this strong sensation present within him for which he had no word. He just knew he didn't like it. But it was there and there was no escape from it.

Peter has reconnected with a very childlike part of himself. He is in touch with early life experience and it seems that it may well be from a time when he had not formulated a language to describe his experiences. It's a time when sensations are present but the language to describe or thinking about those sensations has not been developed. There is present what an adult would term 'sadness', but for a child who does not have the word 'sadness' in their vocabulary they cannot think of it in this way. It is therefore either emerging from a pre-verbal time, or a verbal time when there was not yet developed the complexity of language that would afford Peter the ability to conceptualise in words this particular sensation. He just knows that he doesn't like experiencing what he is experiencing.

Peter was taking a very deep breath. His breathing was not flowing easily; it kind of juddered as he breathed in. Michael felt the urge to reach out to Peter and yet he did not want to interrupt the flow of experiencing. Yet he was also aware that reaching out verbally might not connect if the language wasn't right. He wanted to enable Peter to communicate what was present for him. He wanted to understand, to empathise. But he didn't know what was happening for Peter in the moment. 'Where are you now?' was a question that had taken hold of his thoughts.

'What is happening to Peter?' He spoke softly, he didn't want to sound like an adult seeking some kind of adult explanation, he just wanted to help Peter communicate what was present for him.

'Peter feels …' There was a pause. He looked up and looked Michael straight in the eyes. 'Why doesn't she love me?'

Michael wanted to close his eyes and contain the power of his own emotion that suddenly affected him, and he wanted to reassure Peter that his mother had loved him, though he knew he couldn't do that – maybe she hadn't. He had to stay with the question, he had to empathise with the need to know, and it was hard. He returned the look and sought to express all the tenderness he was feeling towards Peter. He sensed his eyes widening a little and he felt sure his own facial expression was reflecting a degree of sadness. He couldn't help it. It would be false to try to obscure this. The reality was he felt sad. It was sad. He had to be how he was, responding as a human being to a little boy who couldn't understand why it seemed that his mummy didn't love him.

Michael said nothing and yet wanted to say everything. He knew that this was unhelpful. Peter was asking a question directly and needed a response. 'Peter needs to know why his mummy didn't love him.' He was aware as he spoke that he had taken out any sense that she had seemed to not love him.

'She didn't, did she?' Peter was feeling himself shifting away from his experience, coming back into his usual self. It was a slow process, like when you wake up in a dream and watch it slowly fade until you could barely remember what it was about. But he didn't lose the memory with this experience.

Michael felt the atmosphere shifting a little and had noticed that Peter's voice had changed again, sounding more like his adult self once more.

'Seems like you didn't experience her love.'

Peter was shaking his head, and had closed his eyes. He took a deep breath and looked back into Michael's eyes. 'What's happening to me?'

'What do you sense is happening, Peter?' Michael did not want to start introducing his own interpretation of what Peter was going through. He wanted him to make his own sense of his experience, integrate it into himself with his own attached meanings, not those of someone else.

'I feel strangely emotional. I feel sadness, huge sadness.' He had closed his eyes. 'I guess it was there just now but I couldn't describe it.'

'Like you didn't have the language?'

Peter nodded. 'Now I do.' He tightened his lips, taking another deep breath as he did so, an instinctive reaction. He had closed his eyes again. He felt the surge as it welled up inside of him. It felt like a huge wave of sadness rising up from somewhere around his solar plexus; it burned up into his throat and into his eyes. The tears flowed; he couldn't stop them. Wave after wave of sadness erupted inside his body. Michael reached over to Peter and held his hands. Peter gripped him tightly as the force of emotion continued to burst out. So much emotion, so much sadness, so much that he couldn't put into words and really wasn't even trying to. It was like standing in a flood of feeling, like a dam had burst inside himself. He could do nothing to stop the power of what was being released. He could only experience it and wonder whether it would ever stop.

Michael continued to hold Peter's hands. His grip remained firm; every now and then it tightened as another wave of powerful emotion pushed into and through Peter's awareness. Michael spoke softly. 'Let it flow, it's OK to let it flow.'

Peter knew he couldn't do anything to stop it, but it was good to hear Michael's reassuring voice. It seemed distant but he heard it. He tightened his grip.

'Hang in there, Peter, hang in there.'

Peter nodded. He had relaxed his grip slightly once more and was taking a deep breath and swallowing. It seemed as though the emotions were beginning to reduce a little, just a little. He blew his breath out of his mouth, and stared ahead of him before looking back at Michael. 'Thanks.'

'It's OK, take your time. Take your time.'

'Yeah. Shit, that unleashed something.' He was still breathing deeply and blowing his breath out of his mouth each time.

Michael was nodding. He still held Peter's hands. He gave them a gentle squeeze. 'Yes.' He nodded slightly as well.

Peter relaxed his grip; he suddenly felt self-conscious sitting there holding Michael's hands. But he had appreciated the contact. He released his grip and withdrew. He sat back in his chair. He had not been conscious of having moved forward, but he obviously had at some point.

Michael stayed sitting forward for a moment or two longer, and then slowly sat back in his chair.

'She didn't, and maybe doesn't, want me, but she can't, won't let go of me.'

'Mhmm.' Michael didn't want to interrupt, wanted to let Peter find his own words at his own pace to make sense of what he had experienced and whatever was now present for him.

Peter sat, aware of feeling suddenly incredibly tired. He could feel it in his eyes and his whole body just felt so heavy. He yawned. 'Ohh, takes it out of you.'

Michael was nodding. 'Burned up a lot of energy just then.'

He yawned again, lifting his hands over his face as he did so and rubbing his eyes. He looked at the clock; the session was nearly due to end.

'I really have been carrying some strong feelings, haven't I?'

Michael nodded.

'Hmm.' Peter paused. 'I'm feeling calm again. Feels like the storm has passed, for now at any rate.'

'Mhmm.'

'Yeah.' He took another deep breath which triggered another yawn. He blinked, trying to clear the tiredness in his eyes.

'Take your time, Peter, you've just had an incredibly powerful experience. You really did connect with something deep and powerful, but you don't need me to tell you that.'

'I know. I'm left with that question, "why didn't she love me?", and that's jumbled into my wonder now why she can't seem to let go of me, even thought she criticises me. It's all so confusing.'

'It isn't easy, it does feel confusing.'

'Good to know I'm not the only one.'

Michael hadn't actually intended to communicate that he felt confused – in fact he didn't – he had been trying to empathise with Michael's confusion. But he decided not to try and explain this, and then get into perhaps saying why he didn't feel confused. He let it go.

'There's a lot to make sense of.'

Peter had tightened his lips as a thought struck him quite forcibly. 'I've got to talk to her, haven't I? I mean, I've got to try and understand, try and find out.'

'Mhmm, what, talk to her to try and make sense of it all?'

'I can only see it from my perspective, I need to know hers. I need to know why. I need to know what happened, why didn't she love me, why didn't she want me. And whether I'm even right about this. Maybe she did love me but couldn't show it?' As he said that he knew that was a hope he was clinging to.

'Mhmm, so much to clarify. Did she love you, did she want you, was she experiencing feelings for you that she couldn't communicate.'

'I need to talk to her, and that won't be easy. I'm sure she'll avoid it somehow, but I must try. But I need to think about it first, and maybe discuss it with you next time, perhaps.' He paused, wondering what he would say and realising he didn't know. He could just see his mother finding a way of avoiding it, or of turning it around and making some critical point from it. But he knew he had to try.

'I'm going to try and say something this week. I'm not sure how or when, but I have to. I'll give it a few days to settle down inside myself.'

The time was up, and the session ended. Peter sat for a few minutes in the car before driving away. Part of him wanted to go home and say something then and there; part of him wanted to go and see Melanie. He couldn't decide. The more he thought about it, the more he felt the need to say something to his mother, and not to delay. But he desperately wanted to see Melanie as well. He was still undecided as he drove away. Fifteen minutes later he was pulling up outside where Melanie lived.

Counselling session 9: 'What is love?', the client reacts to questioning

27 October

Peter spoke to Melanie after the last session, and had then headed home. He'd called his mother to say he was going to be later than planned. She'd somewhat reluctantly accepted it. Peter had ended up spending more time with Melanie than he had planned, though he did return home around 9.30pm. By then he had decided not to say anything to her. But he knew he would have to at some point. He was tired. The counselling session had taken it out of him.

Now he was sitting in the car outside Michael's house, reflecting on his week. He still hadn't spoken to his mother. He just couldn't. Something kept stopping him, holding him back. He sort of knew that logically he needed to take that step, but he never did. It left him angry and frustrated, but he contained it, at least, he thought he did. He hadn't fully appreciated that his irritability was being noticed at work.

Five minutes later and he was in the counselling room with Michael, and he had begun by describing his reaction to the previous session. 'I talked a lot to Melanie, I guess I was re-running what had happened, and it came up a couple more times during the week when I was with her. But I can't say anything at home. I want to and yet . . .'

'It doesn't sound like ambivalence, sounds like you want to say something but there is something else within you that currently stops you.'

'Am I ambivalent? Doesn't feel like it and yet it must look like it.' Peter thought some more. 'It's not that I don't want to say anything, I do, but I can't.'

'Mhmm, you want to but you cannot.' Michael waited to see what direction Peter would take.

He took a deep breath and spoke on the outbreath. 'I don't know. I sometimes don't feel much like a man.' The words had come out almost before Peter knew what he had been saying, but they did capture a feeling that he had sometimes.

'Don't feel much like a man?' Michael's questioning tone invited Peter to explore his feelings.

'Well, I mean, I should be able to say something, you know?'

'Mhmm, feels like you should.' Michael didn't add the fact that he couldn't; that was not where Peter's current focus was.

'I should be able to. I mean, and then as I think that, part of me wants to forget it, let it go, not make a fuss. All these excuses come into my head, justifying my inaction. So many reasons not to say anything.'

'I guess there must be quite a list of reasons that you experience.' Michael sought to empathise but use different words, perhaps to encourage Peter a little further into engaging with the reasons that were now the focus of the session.

'They're excuses, but it sounds better if I call them reasons.'

'Important for it to sound better?'

Peter could feel himself going quiet as he took on board Michael's response. He didn't like not saying anything, and yet he also wondered at what reaction it would get.

'I mean, what do I say? "Mother, why don't you love me?" I can't say that.'

'OK, so "Mother, why don't you love me" isn't the way you want to say it.'

Peter was shaking his head. He could still feel a kind of cold silence inside himself, like a creeping numbness in the pit of his stomach. And his head felt a bit like it was full of cotton wool, but it was somehow compacted and heavy. His eyes were suddenly feeling gritty.

Peter tightened his lips and looked down. He closed his eyes and tried to think, but it was like his brain wasn't working. He just felt himself sitting with a kind of blank space between his ears. He looked up and across to Michael. Michael seemed so patient, just listened. Reminded him a bit of his father, that kind of passive way of being. It kind of irritated him as well. His father hadn't been much help when he'd been alive, so what the hell use was Michael going to be, sitting there making these fine responses to whatever he said. But did it get him anywhere? Did it give him answers? Daft bastard, at least that was what Peter found himself thinking. He caught himself and felt quite shocked that his thoughts had strayed in the way that they had. That wasn't how he thought of Michael, who he felt had been so helpful, had really helped him uncover some things about his past. But the feelings he had just had, they had been quite strong. He kept his thoughts to himself.

'So, what do I say?'

'You want someone to tell you what to say?'

Michael has avoided the trap of trying to tell Peter what to say. Instead, his empathic question has kept the focus on Peter and allows him to develop a clearer appreciation of what his needs are.

Peter kind of moved his head from side to side. 'Well, no, not so much what to say, more how to say it.'

'How to say ...' Michael deliberately tailed off his sentence to see if it provoked a reaction from Peter.

'How to say,' he shook his head, 'I don't know … how to say, where were you, I guess. Why did you react against me? Why have I never felt loved?'

'Why have you never felt loved.' Michael noted that this was a definite shift of emphasis, away from the blaming attitude of why didn't you love me, to more ownership of the experience of not feeling loved. Quite a sophisticated distinction. Michael put his thoughts aside and waited for Peter to continue.

Peter had raised his arms and rubbed his hands through his hair, bringing them back down on to his cheeks. 'Do I feel loved?' A look of puzzlement had appeared on his face and Michael noticed it.

'You look puzzled at that, at ''Do you feel loved?'' '

'I was suddenly struck with the wonder if I know what it feels like to be loved. I mean, how do you know? How do I know if what I feel is to do with feeling loved? I mean, well, I don't know what I mean.' Peter felt lost in his words. He was frowning. He was thinking of Melanie. He thought he loved her. He was sure he loved her. But did he? Was it love? And did she love him? Did she? He thought so. He thought that was what he felt, but what did he feel? He suddenly felt quite anxious. 'I don't think I know what love is, Michael, and that feels really uncomfortable.'

'What is love, and not knowing, not being sure, leaves a feeling of discomfort or unease maybe?' Michael spoke slowly and calmly, holding the focus on the not knowing and the discomfort. He held steady eye contact with Peter as he spoke. He wanted to create a space, a period for Peter to allow what he had said to sink in, for him to connect with it. It seemed important, hugely important. Peter was questioning not only whether he had been loved, but also whether he had felt love and now whether he knew how to recognise it, how to know what it is.

'I don't think I really know. But I think I'm learning.' He smiled. He was thinking of Melanie and of the sweet moments they shared together. That felt like love, a sort of warm tickly sensation in his stomach, or somewhere around there, and a kind of pressure, a sort of swollen sensation in his heart. He was taking a deep breath as he thought about these things and he could suddenly smell Melanie's perfume. It was so clear, so sharp and yet quite subtle. He was shaking his head slightly as he continued. 'I love her, I'm sure of it. And it's so new. I've never felt like this before, never.'

'So, you love her, and it's a new experience.' Michael guessed Peter was talking about Melanie, at least he could really see that he was talking about his mother, but he didn't know. He let Peter continue, hoping he would clarify it rather than perhaps cutting across Peter's process by asking him to clarify.

'I think it is. It's just so, so … oh I don't know, she fills me up. I just feel like I want to breathe her into my body. What's that about? I don't know. I don't need to know.' As Peter stopped speaking he realised he suddenly felt awkward and embarrassed. He'd never talked like this to anyone before and he was suddenly feeling that somehow it wasn't right to talk like this, not to another man. It wasn't sort of what you did, talk in this way. And yet …

Michael noticed that Peter had coloured up a bit.

'Feels kind of difficult, embarrassing talking like this?'

Peter nodded. 'Yes, I mean, well, but I have to, I mean, I need someone else to know about how I feel. I can't tell mother, she, well, I don't think she'd want to know. It does feel good talking about this but I still don't know. Is it love? What is love?' He paused. 'What *is* love?'

'What does love mean to you, Peter?' Michael wasn't sure if he was being directive. It wasn't that he was taking Peter's focus away from the theme. Maybe he should have simply reflected back the words in the same tone of voice and left Peter to choose his response. And yet he couldn't deny his own curiosity. Given what he knew about Peter, and about his background and early life experience, he was intrigued to hear what Peter had to say, and to help him explore his inner world of trying to make sense of love.

Probably a supervision issue to explore why Michael's curiosity is so strong as to cause him to word his response in the way that he did. A simple 'what is love' empathic response could have been enough. The person-centred counsellor will want to remain within the client's inner world and yet there may be occasions when congruence demands them to voice something of themselves. Is Michael speaking with full awareness of why he is responding in the way that he has, or is there an unrecognised need driving his curiosity that might make this particular element of the encounter less than therapeutic?

Peter sat and thought. Michael's question had made a quite distinct impact on him. His wondering about what love is had felt kind of gentle and now it seemed like he was being asked a question that demanded an answer. Yet he knew he did not have an answer. That was precisely the point. He didn't know, so what was Michael asking him? He felt frustrated; he felt like something had been lost.

'I've lost it. Your question has somehow taken it away?'

'Taken it away?' Michael was really unsure what was happening. He felt suddenly disconnected from Peter, unsure what he was talking about. He noted his reaction and guessed that something had happened for him to feel this way. 'I felt like I was just, I don't know, drifting into what love is all about and your question pulled me up. Felt like I had to have an answer, that it had to mean something to me. But I don't know what it is. I don't know.' Peter had raised his voice.

Michael sensed that the reaction was likely to be in part the result of his question but that it could also be frustration and anger linked to his past experience – or lack of experience – of love. He noted that there could be a temptation to become defensive. Yes, in part he was being attacked, and maybe justifiably so. No need to go there. There may be time to come back to that later. 'Yes, my question took you away from what you were experiencing.'

Peter could feel anger inside himself, 'always bloody questions' was what he found himself thinking. He was fed up with questions. He'd felt good talking just now, but now, well, now was different. It wasn't that he was reflecting on the difference, it was simply there, he was in another place in himself, an angry place, fed up with having to find answers. But was it OK to be angry here? Was it? He wasn't sure, but he knew he felt like he wanted to say something more forcefully. He stared down and felt his jaw tighten.

Michael felt uncomfortable. He knew that his response had taken Peter into whatever he was currently experiencing, and yet, at the same time, he also wanted to trust that maybe this was what needed to happen.

While this justification for directing a client into a fresh area of his inner world might be made, that it was simply part of the process to which the therapist had unwittingly contributed, there is danger in this. How can we be sure that it is therapeutic? How can we be definite that what has been said is a congruent voicing of something that has relevance for the therapeutic relationship, and not simply the therapist pursuing their own curiosity or, in other exchanges, perhaps expressing a defensiveness through directing a client into an area of their life that the therapist feels most comfortable with?

For the person-centred counsellor, the need for accurate self-awareness is vitally important. The counsellor from this discipline will be using themselves, will be monitoring their own reactions and, at times, making judgements as to whether urges to speak or behave in certain ways have relevance to the therapeutic process, or are simply their own 'stuff' needing an exploration in supervision or in therapy. The importance of congruence is such a key aspect to person-centred working that accurate experiencing of their own inner world is a crucial element in successful person-centred counselling.

Michael also recognised that he couldn't just brush it aside and justify what he had said. And yet, at the time, it had felt reasonable. He waited for Peter to respond. He had noticed his jaw tighten and that he was now looking down. He somehow looked less relaxed, or rather, to place emphasis where it would be a more accurate reflection of how he was experiencing Peter, more stressed.

Peter was pursing his lips. Should he say something? He was really struggling to be able to give himself permission, and he wasn't at all sure why. So he continued to sit, angry and uncomfortable.

Michael was feeling uncomfortable as well. He knew that he could feel uncomfortable when clients were reacting to him, he'd been there before, but he wasn't totally sure whether he was uncomfortable with himself or with Peter's reaction – or both. It felt appropriate to own it. He wondered exactly what was happening for Peter as well and decided to voice this.

'Leaves me feeling uncomfortable suddenly and I'm wondering what reaction you have.'

Peter looked up. 'Cut off.'

'Cut off?' Michael was aware that he was frowning slightly, unsure what Peter was meaning.

'Yes. Like I was trying to say something and then it all goes, dismissed, taken out.'

Michael nodded and was thinking back to what had occurred previously. Had he cut off Peter with his question about what love meant to him? What had happened in that moment? If anything it seemed like he had taken the general question of 'what is love?', which Peter had voiced, and made it personal. So making it personal, had that caused the sense of being cut off? He didn't know. Tempting to ask, he thought, but another question, and he knew he needed to stay with Peter.

'What you said was dismissed by me.' Michael didn't voice it as a question, but as a statement. Seemed stronger, and got away from the questioning pattern that they had slipped into these last few minutes.

Peter nodded. 'And I hate that.'

'Mhmm, I hear that, you hate being dismissed.'

Peter was taking a deep breath, still full of discomfort, anger, generally feeling tight in himself. He had an image in his head of a time when his father was alive, when he had come home late for dinner one evening – been out with friends – must have been about 14. He was late because the train had been cancelled. He didn't know till they'd got to the station. Got home and his mother had gone for him, asking questions, kept asking questions and having a go at him. And he had no answer. The train had been cancelled. What could he have done? She wouldn't accept it. All she seemed concerned about was his dinner which had dried up in the oven after all the time she'd spent preparing it. And it wasn't that it had been that much, all that fuss over . . . he realised he couldn't remember what had been cooked. Didn't matter. Just remembered she wouldn't listen. He remembered looking over to his father who had just shrugged and gone back to watching the TV. It hadn't been the only occasion when he'd felt dismissed, not listened to, barraged with questions he didn't have an answer to, or rather, as in this case, he had an answer but it wasn't acceptable.

Michael sat watching Peter as the silence between them continued. He wasn't feeling so uncomfortable now, having said what he had said before and owned his discomfort. And he recognised how important it was for Peter to feel heard, listened to. He could only guess how often he had not been heard and what impact that must have had in shaping his structure of self. Not good enough to be listened to. Not worthy enough to have your view accepted about things.

These are classic ways in which an individual will interpret this kind of experience. It could be a one-off experience, but in a highly charged and significant context, or it might occur over time, but either way the person is left feeling less of a person in some way, and not valued. This leads to the person creating a particular view of themselves which they may then live out and seek, through their behaviour, to reinforce. At the same time, powerful feelings may be present, feelings that were unexpressed when these 'introjects' were being established. So, for instance, unvoiced anger at not being listened to can leave the person with what a client might describe as an 'angry me' sense of self that emerges when the experience is repeated. Or there might be present a 'make myself invisible' urge if the way that the person learned to deal with the situation was to get away, either physically or emotionally, from the situation.

What is important to recognise is the uniqueness of the individual, that they will attribute meanings to experiences that will be unique to them. Of course, there will be similarities with others, but the process and the effect that a client experiences and then reveals in therapy is theirs. The structure of self is made up of these accepted, discreet conditioned responses and beliefs about oneself. 'Configurations of self' is how they have been described (Mearns). The person-centred counsellor acknowledges that these many identities are each an important part of the client's structure of self and need to be heard and allowed freedom to be present.

There was also an anxiety present within Peter's discomfort and anger – and the anger was more of a frustrated anger. It was a familiar feeling. Often in his life there had times when he had wanted to be different, but had found himself impelled to behave in ways that were all too familiar. Shrinking back from situations was one of these, particularly where he felt he would be putting himself at the centre of attention. He'd lose any composure he might have had. His self-confidence evaporated and he was left simply trying to contain the anxious feelings that became present. He felt anxious now. He knew there were things he wanted to say, and it felt like there was a pressure for him to say something. The silence was feeling uncomfortable to him. He wanted to end it. He had to say something.

'I'm finding this really difficult. Don't know what to say.' He glanced at the clock. Still 20 minutes of the session to run. He'd hoped it would be nearly at an end so he could get away.

'Mhmm. Difficult sitting here with what you are experiencing . . .'

Peter nodded. He felt a million miles away from that love they'd been talking about, and he expressed this. 'What I was talking about feels a million miles away.'

'Million miles away from what you were talking about, now in a very different place in yourself.'

'Some really familiar feelings.'

'Mhmm.' Michael waited to see if Peter would name these feelings. It seemed to be a really sensitive time and he didn't want to push him too fast. Rather let him disclose at his own pace, if that is what he wants or needs to do.

'And I do feel irritated, and frustrated at not feeling heard. I've got a lot of memories that come back to me about times when I haven't been heard as a child, like I said, feeling dismissed. Used to get questions, questions, questions as a child. Could never be good enough for her. And now it feels like, well, feels like it's the same here.'

'Too many questions, and not feeling heard?'

Peter shook his head. 'No, I do feel heard. Of course I feel heard here, but, well, just now, the place where I was felt so precious somehow and it's gone.'

'And it went when I specifically asked you that question?'

'Yes, about what love meant to me, and something happened. I was in touch with my feelings for Melanie, and they really are beautiful feelings.' He could feel his eyes becoming moist as he was speaking. 'And then all this other stuff.'

'Your love for Melanie *is* precious, it's a really sweet experience, but when I asked the question it seemed to provoke a reaction that took you away from those feelings.'

'It's scary, they went so fast. Like I just went into another place, a place that's familiar. Where I've been all my life – or so it seems. And I'm trying desperately to get away from.'

'So the feelings are familiar, all too familiar, and there is a desperation to get away from them.'

'Get away, be in another place.' He paused before repeating himself, speaking a little more softly as he did so. 'Be in another place. Getting away to another place. But it's new, I mean, really new.' He was looking at Michael now. 'It's precious, fragile, but I need it, it's my way ahead, my salvation – I don't know. But it really is that important, she's that important to me. The contrast between how I feel when I'm with her and when I'm at home is vast.'

Michael, now mindful of the sensitivity within Peter to being asked questions, and not wanting his reaction to this experience to take him away again, responded with simple and direct empathy for the content of what Peter was saying. 'Vast contrast. Such a precious relationship with Melanie, while at home . . .' Michael didn't finish the sentence; he felt he didn't need to.

'While at home . . .' Peter's jaw tightened once again. He shook his head and took a deep breath. 'While at home, well.' Another pause and further shaking of his head. 'I can't breathe there, Michael, I can't breathe. It's suffocating me, but I've been so used to it. I can't believe I deserve something better.' Peter spoke with emotion and was surprised to hear what he had said about not believing he deserved something better.

'Mhmm, all those years have left you feeling that you don't deserve anything better, but now that better has come along.'

'And I don't know what to do, and it's wonderful, and I'm scared of losing it.' Peter had drawn his hands into fists; there was real tension in his body. 'So scared of losing it.'

'So scared of losing the wonderful feelings that you are experiencing.'

Peter nodded and felt his body relax. As he heard Michael speak it was like his whole being was saying, 'yes', and somewhere within him he was aware that there was a doubt. Did he deserve it? Would it last? A seed of doubt, no, more than a seed. He doubted that it was possible but he so wanted it to last. He loved Melanie. He was experiencing feelings he'd never encountered before in his life. And that love was precious and sweet – like drops of honey, and yet more subtle. More like the taste of honey translated into a fragrance. Light and subtle, but how easy it was for his other, heavy, negative feelings to overwhelm him.

'You know, I know I reacted earlier, but I think I've learned a lot from it. I really am carrying some baggage from my past, I really do not see myself as deserving good things. I am sensitive, so sensitive, to not being listened to, put down, being put in situations that I can't cope with – questioned where I can't give an answer that's acceptable.' He'd brought his hand up to his mouth. 'I really am wondering what next? How do I resolve all this? How do I let go and move on? How do I break free of, I don't know what to call it, the *me* that life has made me?'

'Big questions, how to break free from the me that life has made you? And what I'm hearing is that that is precisely what you are doing, but it's a process.'

'I guess so. But I wish it was instant. I wish I could let go of who I am – was – I don't know, who I am I guess. I'm still so full of all the crap from the past.' He paused before continuing, a thought having struck him. 'You know, people say sometimes that emotional abuse is more difficult than physical abuse, and I've always thought that's daft, but now I wonder. Constantly not being valued, not feeling loved – that was the . . . is the really big one. I guess people that experience physical abuse feel that as well. I don't know. I didn't experience that, but the emotional and, I guess, mental battering that it feels I took. Never good enough. Always had to do things her way, what she wanted. And my father, he couldn't cope with it any more than I could. But in a way I saw how it made him. And I don't want to spend my life like that. Melanie's so different to my mother – thank God.' He paused again as another thought came to him. 'I know they say that men look for partners that are like their mothers, but I definitely want one that's totally different, totally opposite.'

A child passing through extreme experiences is likely to carry a dual reaction. Partly he or she will be conditioned into normalising what has occurred and therefore will be seeking to perpetuate it, to maintain the senses of self that have developed within the experience. However, there will be a part that yearns for difference, yearns for another experience. This may stem from what they see others experiencing, giving them a sense that it could be different. Often this part does not get heard, or is unable to assert itself. But it seems to me that it can be present and will have a vital part to play when the person begins to address issues and seeks change. Both aspects of the person are real to them; both have an equal validity as both emerged in reaction to the experiences that occurred in their lives. Where negative conditioning is present the person develops in ways to try and make the best of what has occurred. But it is conditioning.

I believe that people have the potential to be free of these 'conditions of worth' but they need the relational experience based on the qualitative values emphasised within the person-centred approach to encourage this. Fundamental to change, though, is a shift in the person's sense of self such that they can feel not just valued but *valuable*, not just loved but *lovable*, not just wanted but *wantable*. It is this psychological transition that I believe is at the heart of successful therapy.

'You want someone very different, completely opposite in fact?'

'Yes, and I'm finding that now with Melanie and I just hope it lasts.' As he spoke Peter felt a mixture of joy and sadness. He so wanted it to last, and yet . . . Would it? He didn't know. But he had to try. Yes, he was changing, but it was painful and slow and he wanted to be different now.

Michael had looked at the clock. 'Yes, you so want it to last.' It somehow felt as though something was summed up by saying that while at the same time being in a setting that only had a couple of minutes left. 'We've just got a couple of minutes left.'

'Yes, I know. It's been a good session. Not an easy one. More to go and think about. Change. It's not simple, is it, breaking free of patterns, of the past – well, the past is also in the present, isn't it? I've got to make changes.'

A quote from Gandhi had popped into Michael's head as he heard Peter speak, though he couldn't recall exactly the words, something about needing to be the change you want to see in the world. He could see how Peter needed to be the change that he wanted in his own world, and somehow it seemed relevant. He shared it. 'I think it was Gandhi who said we have to be the change we want to see in the world, something like that.'

'Yes, personal responsibility. Down to us, down to me.' He was nodding his head thoughtfully. 'Yes, I have to be the change that I want to see in my world, don't I?'

Michael nodded, pleased that Peter had re-formulated it to reflect his own situation.

The session ended. As he was leaving Peter mentioned that it was Melanie's birthday at the weekend and he was taking her to see *Phantom of the Opera*. Michael had seen it himself some while back, and wondered how they might react to it. He said it was a powerful show and hoped they had a great time together.

Peter walked thoughtfully back to his car. His mind went back over the session. So much to reflect on. So much to break free of. Did he need to talk to his mother, or just get on with his life, with what he wanted? He knew what he wanted – Melanie. At the moment she was his horizon, the only direction he wanted to move in.

Meanwhile Michael had returned back into the counselling room to reflect on the session and write his notes. He kept brief notes of the factual content, but he also wrote about the process sometimes. The latter he didn't keep; he used them as a way to self-process. He felt he needed to after that session, particularly as his response to Peter had had a major impact on him, and yet had contributed a lot to the session. It had helped Peter – and himself – gain greater awareness of the contrasts. He had to be mindful of Peter's sensitivity to questioning – not to avoid it, this had to be encountered and fresh responses developed – and this would occur as Peter himself changed. It did all seem quite fragile and yet there seemed to be a purpose as well. Peter really wanted to change and he had someone in his life that he wanted to change for. Did he want to change for Melanie or for himself? Could they be distinguished? He'd heard it said so many times that if you are going to change, you have to do it for yourself, not in order to achieve a particular response from someone else. He didn't know. He didn't like statements that were generalised and didn't take into account the specific experiences of an individual.

He knew that within Peter there was present that 'actualising tendency' urging greater fulfilment and satisfaction. Peter had discovered an area in his life, and in himself, that was satisfying a huge need – to love and feel loved. How that would develop, he did not know, but it seemed to him that Peter was in exactly the right set of circumstances for change to occur. *Phantom of the Opera*, that would be interesting. What would he make of that? He realised he was really looking forward to the next session, and also aware that he mustn't let his own experience dominate, or ask too many questions just to feed his own curiosity. He was smiling. Therapy. Life. Circumstances. One vast process leading us ... God knows where. He was in a very reflective place. We work as therapists with the particular, the individuals, with the specifics, and yet we are all it seems bound up in some vaster process that seemed to be – well, it was what he believed – something about finding ways of bringing more goodness into the world by finding that goodness in ourselves. He wasn't sure how that fitted into person-centred theory, but it was a fundamental belief that he had. And for Michael, that goodness started with creating right relationship, healthy relationship, relationships that empowered, that offered the opportunity for a collaborative spirit to be present. Love.

Points for discussion

- How did you feel Michael handled the cathartic release? Were there occasions when, as the counsellor, you might have responded or behaved differently?
- What has love got to do with human development and the counselling process? What does love mean to you?
- How would you have felt had a client reacted as Peter did to Michael's question about love? How would you have dealt with it?
- Evaluate the last two sessions from the standpoint of applying person-centred theory.
- What issues would you take to supervision from these two sessions, why, and what would you be hoping for from supervision?
- Write your notes for these two sessions.

CHAPTER 7

Counselling session 10: learning to feel loved

3 November

'Hi Peter, come on in.'

'Thanks. It's turned cold again.'

'Yes. Come on through.' Michael followed Peter to the counselling room. Peter took off his coat and hung it behind the door, and sat down. He had a lot to talk about and was really quite excited at the prospect of talking his experiences through with Michael.

'So, where do you want to begin today, Peter?'

'It's been, well,' Peter shook his head, 'it's been quite a week. Very much centred around the weekend.'

Michael nodded, but did not say anything, allowing Peter to continue at his own pace and without interruption.

'You know I said that we were going to see *Phantom of the Opera?*'

Michael nodded. 'Yes, you mentioned it as you were leaving last week.'

'Well, we did.' He was shaking his head. 'Have you seen it?'

'A while back.'

'What did you think about it?'

Michael didn't want to get drawn into his experience, but he wanted to be open and honest and respond to Peter. 'Powerful, very powerful.' He kept his response brief and waited for Peter to say more.

'Yes, it was for me too. Well, for us, but particularly for me.' He was shaking his head. 'It just really got to me, touched something so deep inside myself.'

Michael nodded and waited.

'I mean, the production was great, all the effects. Always amazes me how people design things like that. But, well, it just,' he shrugged, 'it just spoke to me. Left me really choked.'

'Mhmm, choked.'

Peter could feel himself back in the theatre. They'd got good seats, a clear view of the stage and all that was happening. 'Just so powerful, it really affected me.' Peter could feel his eyes watering as he spoke, and his throat felt like it had a lump in it. 'Something about – no, so much about – the phantom that just resonated with me. I mean, not that I have his problems, and yet, somehow, there was something similar.'

'Something similar, something resonated . . .' Michael didn't respond with a question but acknowledged the presence of a 'something'.

'The bit when his history comes out, being taken round in a cage for people to see because of his disfigurement, and how it left him feeling angry, wanting some kind of a revenge I guess, at least that's how it seemed to me, and yet, and yet, he was offering something so sweet through his music, and his capacity to love, to want to love, and to be loved. His yearning but having to wear a mask to hide his face.' He was shaking his head. 'We all wear masks, don't we, hiding parts of ourselves from others. Even from ourselves sometimes.'

'Mhmm.' Michael wasn't sure where Peter was heading, and he didn't need to know. His job was to stay with him, listen and let him know that he had heard, accept warmly whatever Peter had and was experiencing, and be accurately in touch with his own inner flow of experience and response.

'Yeah. Something about being treated the way he was, and how it made him become the person he then became. And the complexity of it all, and yet a simplicity as well.'

Michael wasn't sure what Peter meant. 'I'm not sure I understand what you mean, the complexity and the simplicity?'

'The horrible experiences he must have gone through that shaped his view of himself, and of others, and of the world. People must have been awful towards him. Imagine his childhood? Mine was, well, almost said heavenly. I mean, it wasn't, but it sort of puts things in perspective, you know?'

Michael nodded. 'Mhmm, fresh perspective.' He waited for Peter to continue.

'Sitting there, I just felt this overwhelming sadness, I mean, really overwhelming. I sat with tears running down my cheeks in that theatre. I was in another place. I've never been affected quite like that. So sad. It just felt so real, so close, so much part of me in some way.'

'What you were feeling was part of you? The sadness, so real, so close.'

'I knew that sadness. It was mine. It was his. I just . . .' He swallowed. 'It's got to me again.' Michael nudged the box of tissues towards Peter who took one out and wiped his eyes.

'The sadness . . .' Peter had brought both his hands up and was holding the sides of his face. 'And yet, deep within that sadness there was a beauty, his singing, his voice, it was like even in spite, or maybe because, of what had happened to him, there was this wonderful voice. But the pain, the hurt, the passion, the intensity. The capacity of a human being to feel and express these things. It just, well, overwhelmed me.' He paused. 'And it wasn't pity.'

'You didn't feel pity?'

Peter shook his head. 'No, I think because I saw the beauty, the incredible passion, but the sadness, the immense sadness of it all. No, not pity. Compassion, yes, and that was great to be put in touch with that feeling. We could do with more compassion in the world. But, yes, my heart went out. But it also left me thinking about myself as well, not directly at the time, thoughts about me kind of came and went, but afterwards, when I really talked about it with Melanie,

I really felt the connection. It was like I kind of recognised the phantom in me. I have anger about how I was treated. I have a form of, I guess, emotional disfigurement. I wear a mask, although I've never really thought of it like that, just thought of it as being me. Like I created a mask and became that mask and forgot who I really was, although I hadn't really forgotten? And that's why it is so complex. And yet the simplicity, that's the beauty, the compassion, the feelings that one human being can have for another.'

Peter stopped speaking. He was taking a deep breath, aware of the immense wave of emotion that was present within him. It felt like it filled his chest and left his arms strangely numb and yet slightly tingly.

'So, a sense that you have a phantom within you, that you wear or have become a mask, that it's all so complex and yet there is a simplicity as well in the human response.' Michael hoped he had captured what Peter had said. He added, 'Is that capturing your experience?'

'Yes, and yet they're just words. It goes beyond words, you know?'

Michael did and his nodding response was genuine.

'I mean, yes, the powerful emotions that the phantom felt. How his life, his attitude towards himself and others was shaped. How he wanted to be in control as well. You know, that was something that struck me. He wanted to control that theatre. He wanted his own opera. But he wanted control. How he must have yearned for that when he was caged and exhibited, when he had all control taken away from him.' Peter went quiet for a few moments. Michael respected it. It seemed to him a silence that needed to be held. 'Control. Not sure how much I've felt in control, and yet somehow I wonder now if that's why I do the work that I do. I mean, computer programming, writing software, it's about being in control, about making things happen the way you want them to happen. I thought about this later, it's like my work is about being in control of a process. I can make things happen a certain way. And I can be sure that what I create will happen the way I want it to. I have control. I've kind of got the idea in my head that this part of the job is actually really important. I need to feel in control.'

'Mhmm. Control, you need to feel in control and your work allows this.'

'Control at work but controlled at home. And I'm going to change that. Melanie and I are going to live together. At least, we are making plans to do this. Haven't told mother yet, but I will do, I have to.'

'So, taking control.'

Peter nodded. His thoughts had gone back to the theatre again. 'Just so much for me from that experience. And I think it came at the right time. What we'd been talking about, coming here, meeting Melanie, it all seemed to be happening at the right time.'

'Uh-uh, everything coming together . . .'

'. . . making me change, creating an opportunity for change. But it's up to me to take it.'

'Yes, up to you.'

'Another thing as well, and I can't remember exactly, but there was something that the woman – Christine, who was the main female character – she says to the phantom that it's not so much his physical disfigurement that concerns her as the effect it has had on his soul. I heard that. It troubled me. It still does. At that really deep level – and I know soul can mean all kinds of things to different people – but the thought that these kinds of disfiguring processes – not just physical, but emotional and mental – can really touch into and affect your soul. I like to believe that somewhere deep in myself is a part of me that is good, that is free of the crap, and yet that line left me unsettled. Does it go that deep? Left me wondering, if that was the case, what hope was there? And then, well, at the end, the passion, the beauty in the singing, there has to be something pure inside us, something that is just untouched and untainted by the horrible things that happen in the world.'

Michael was deeply touched by the passion in Peter's voice as he had been speaking. These were matters that really mattered to him, that went to the core, that were rooted in his heart. He wanted to acknowledge this.

Empathy is not only about conveying back to the client an appreciation of the words that he or she has used, or of the meaning that those words convey. Sometimes it has to go further, and embrace the passion, the drive, the experience that is present behind the words communicated.

'I hear the passion in your voice, Peter, these are matters that go to the very core of your being.'

'They do. I want to believe that there is something good and beautiful. Yes, horrible, unspeakable things are done in our world. Makes me shiver at the thought of it. The human capacity to inflict pain on others – and then get pleasure from it. Argghh. Horrible. But it happens, and continues to happen. And yet, within all that people can somehow find something deeper – sometimes, not all the time. The phantom brought beauty into the world through his music, his song. But people couldn't see beyond his face. Maybe he couldn't, I don't know, but the capacity for beauty was there.'

'The capacity for beauty in spite of the horribleness of what can happen.'

'Here am I, masked up by my past, caged up in myself by the rejection and lack of love that was inflicted on me, angry, frustrated, wanting to break out but seemingly powerless to do so. I was going to say impotent. It felt like that, looking back, like I'd been rendered impotent. And yet – well, one thing I know from my relationship with Melanie is that I am certainly not impotent. And after the theatre trip, we had the most wonderful night together.'

Michael felt such a wonderful warm glow inside himself as he heard Peter speak. 'Maybe the mask is crumbling, you're realising parts of yourself that you did not believe were there. I feel really good about what you are saying, it really gives me a warm glow hearing you speak about the wonderful and fulfilling and exciting experiences you are having.'

Peter was really grateful to Michael for saying that. It somehow felt hugely important. Knowing that it was having that effect, that another person was feeling good about what was happening for him. 'Thanks, that means a lot to me.'

Sometimes it is important for a client to know that what affects them also affects others – the good feelings and experiences and those that are more painful. It is validating for the client, giving a sense that what they are experiencing is perhaps more alive, more real. When a client talks about something that deeply moves or affects the counsellor, the person-centred approach will encourage that the effect is made visible, that there is transparency. Letting genuinely human reactions be out in the open encourages them to be more fully present. Permission is given for feelings to be felt. The client may be enabled to openly express what they are experiencing, to be who and what they are, without screening, and without raising a mask.

Michael nodded but said nothing, wanting to leave it open for Peter to pick up the threads and take the exploration where he needed to.

'So, it's all made a big impression on me. I really do feel different. I came away from that theatre with so much going on for me. And I wanted to talk about it and I wanted to be silent as well, both at the same time. Crazy. But it was like it filled me up with so much. And at the same time, it wasn't just filling me up, but making me aware, making me aware of how I was feeling, of what I was about.'

Again, the urgency, the passion in his voice. Michael was so heartened to hear Peter speaking this way. Yes, something had changed, and profoundly so. Whether it would last, well, what did that mean? The only reality is the present, and the present has changed insofar as Peter's experience of it. 'Making you aware of what you are about. Seems to sum it up somehow, and yet it is so much more than those few words, isn't it?'

'Much more, and yet it is about that. There are some spooky things with mirrors in that production, and I wasn't totally clear on what it all meant, but I do feel like maybe in some way I can see myself a little more clearly now. I can't really, completely put it into words. But there is a difference. I feel ...' He thought about it. 'I think I feel more assured somehow, more self-assured. It's like, yes, it's like I've lost some kind of anxiety? Not sure if that's the right word for it though. But an edge, a kind of unsettledness. Yes, not so unsettled by it all. It's like I have a direction and I'm a little clearer about the me that is taking that direction, and they're both connected – bit of a chicken and egg situation. Direction is clearer because I am clearer, but I am clearer because the direction is clearer. And it doesn't matter which came first.' He paused. 'Maybe chicken and egg is the wrong analogy, but I know what I mean.'

'Let me check that I understand what you mean. You feel a little clearer about who you are, and about where you are wanting to go, and that the two processes are connected.'

A useful way of wording a need to clarify what has been said. It conveys to the client that the counsellor is listening but wants to understand.

'I think I'd say they're one process. And it feels exciting. Yes, there is a certain scariness – that's too strong a word – but I don't want to say anxiety. Just has a kind of edge to it, and that's OK, because of how I'm feeling about things.'

'So, excitement, and an edge but not what you'd want to call anxiety, and one process.'

Peter nodded. 'I really went to that – I don't know, it's not opera, is it a musical, what do you call it? Anyway, seeing *Phantom* has come at the right time, I know it, I can feel it. And I think for both of us. Melanie got a lot from it as well. She could see herself in some of the characters, but not to the degree that I identified with aspects of the phantom. And it has helped her understand me because it helped me to become more in touch and open. And we need that. So, yes, what a night. What a night.' Peter's thoughts had shifted back to the period afterwards. So much love. He'd felt so much love for her. He suddenly felt very quiet and very grateful for what he had in his life. And he realised that it was a new feeling for him. Or was it something he was just experiencing more sharply, or more completely in some way? 'You know, I've got good things in my life. I suddenly feel very grateful.' And as he spoke he burst into tears as a surge of emotion ripped through him, completely taking him, and Michael, by surprise.

Michael reached over and held Peter's wrist. Peter moved his hand so that they were holding hands. He gripped Michael. He wasn't in a place to make sense of what he was experiencing; he was simply affected by the feelings that were present within him. Melanie was very much part of his experience. He suddenly realised he knew something, something that he'd sort of known, but was all of a sudden really known. He swallowed and took another tissue. 'Ohh,' and blew out a breath. He took a moment to regain a bit of composure as what he wanted to say he knew was going to bring more emotion with it. But he had to say it. He had to. 'It's like,' he paused, and swallowed, the emotions were close to breaking through again, 'it's like I'd begun to know that I was loved – by Melanie – but it has been in my head.' He swallowed again and took a deep breath. 'But I think that now, and for the first time in a long time, maybe ever, I think I'm beginning to know what it *feels* like to be loved.' He closed his eyes as they suddenly watered again and he felt the emotion hit his solar plexus. 'I've learned to feel love, and I think I'm now learning to feel *loved*.' His grip on Michael's hand tightened once more. Michael returned the grip. So much was communicated through that empathic response, more than could be put into words. This was male solidarity, two men connecting with a deep and profound human experience – the experience of feeling loved. Michael knew this feeling; he'd gone on his own journey into this experience in the past and could appreciate the power and overwhelming nature for what was occurring for Peter. He was ready to give him a hug, but stayed with the contact they already had.

Peter's grip lessened. Michael adjusted his own grip.

Peter took a deep breath; in fact they both did. Silence descended on them. The eye contact was steady. Deep communication was present though no words were passed between them. There was no thought either, just two men, connecting in some profound way, some kind of male solidarity in the need to feel loved. The outer silence continued. Yet at some deeper level it seemed as though there was no separation, no 'I and thou', but a place of communion, a place where individual identity dissolves into something else, and yet remains as well. A place where identity extends and expands beyond the personal, and yet includes it. There was nothing to say because somehow both knew.

It was Peter who spoke first. He spoke softly. 'Thank you.'

'Thank you too. I think we have both gained from this experience.'

Peter nodded. 'I feel . . .' he paused, 'I don't really want to talk about how I feel, I just want to be with it.'

Michael nodded. 'Sure, I can appreciate that. Take your time.'

'Thanks.' Peter broke eye contact and looked away. He wanted to be with himself. He had no thoughts for what had just occurred, but he knew it had been profound, and he knew it was timely. He was aware the session was soon to end and he wanted to just sit quietly. So he sat, silently being with himself, feeling a wonderful warm calmness, a kind of reassurance that all was well and would be well. He hadn't ever experienced anything quite like it. Like something was telling him, 'it's OK'. And he knew that all was OK. Yes, he had problems in his life, but they somehow didn't matter quite the same. All would be well. It was like he had touched a place in himself that knew a kind of secret, something that most of the time people were blind to. He didn't want to go, he didn't want to move, just wanted to stay in this place. It wasn't that he felt high; it wasn't that kind of sudden rush upwards. He hadn't gone up, it was more about going within, going deep, not a high. But it was definitely good. He blinked and moved his head. He was aware as he moved his body and came back into awareness of the sensations within it that his back was stiff. He stretched and as he did so could feel something of what he had been experiencing fading. Yet the calmness remained.

'Time to head off. I don't want to talk about this, not just at the moment. Feel I want to just be with it, take it with me.'

'Sure.' They confirmed the next appointment. As they stood up, Peter felt the urge to reconnect with Michael, he felt a natural instinct to shake his hand, and while that hand-to-hand contact they had had earlier had felt so profound, now it didn't seem enough. It felt awkward and formal. He needed it to be more personal. 'I think I need to give you a hug.'

Michael smiled and opened his arms. The two men stood, holding each other. Not tightly, but firmly. The earlier feelings echoed between them once more, though not to such depth. Michael had decided to stay in the position until Peter was ready to release. He wanted Peter to feel in control, to be in his own process for as long as he needed. It was about 30 seconds or so, maybe a little longer, when Peter released his grip and stepped back. 'Thanks again. I'm not sure what has happened, but it feels good, it feels right, I feel different, and I want to take this with me into my week, and into my relationship with Melanie. And maybe it'll affect how I am at home and at work. We'll see.'

Michael nodded. 'Have a good week. We can talk it through next time if you want to, or whatever else comes up for you.'

'Thanks.'

Peter headed out the door and Michael went and sat back down to process his experience. He was aware of feeling different. He'd had some profound experiences himself, both as a client and as a therapist, but what had just occurred somehow seemed very powerful, more so than what he had experienced before. And yet he also was aware that it was something he was finding hard to think about, as though the experience went beyond thinking. It was like thought couldn't capture it, and neither could emotion. He was also experiencing a calmness and couldn't really get hold of the experience in his mind. It was like it was something that had emerged within the therapeutic process beyond day-to-day words, thoughts and feelings. He began to write his notes. They were very brief. He put them aside, deciding that he might add to them later. He didn't feel in the place to write much. He decided he needed to go and sit for a while in a space away from the counselling room. He went out to the kitchen; one of the other therapists was there making a cup of tea. He joined her. He only said he'd had a powerful session, didn't go into any detail, respecting client confidentiality. They chatted about this and that. Throughout, though, Michael knew that he was still with his experience with Peter. He had another client in 10 minutes and decided he needed to go out for a couple of minutes of fresh air, and then he'd still have a few minutes to compose himself.

Points for discussion

- How has this session left you feeling?
- How is the actualising tendency finding expression within Peter?
- What were the key moments in this session?
- Evaluate Michael's responses. Was the person-centred approach consistently applied?
- What would you take to supervision from this session if you had been the counsellor?
- Write notes for this session.

Supervision session 3

4 November

'I really need to talk about what is happening with Peter. I am concerned that I may be struggling to keep myself clear to be accurately responsive to him.'
'OK. What's on your mind?'
'Well, I've seen him three times since our last session. The first of those three he reconnected with himself as a little boy not feeling loved by his mother, really confused about why she didn't love him. The theme of love was clearly a big one, and is – it carried into the next session, though then, as I recall, more linked to pondering on the nature of love in the context of his relationship

with his girlfriend, Melanie. He was really expressing, quite beautifully, his feelings for her and then was questioning the meaning of love in a quite general way. And then I responded in a way that really impacted on him and our relationship for the rest of the session.'

'Go on. What happened?'

'Well, I made the question of love more specific, I remember asking something like, "So what does love mean to you?" At least, I think that's how I worded it. I jotted down what I thought I'd said after the session. Anyway, it really put a block on Peter, and he really struggled with it. He later revealed how he had felt dismissed, not listened to, that it was linked back to his childhood experiences. It really pushed him into a difficult place in himself.'

'So you have a feeling of pushing him somewhere that was really uncomfortable. How was that for you?'

'I wasn't at ease either. Part of me wanted to say to myself, "hey, it's OK, it's just part of the process", but in truth I don't think it was necessarily helpful in that moment. Peter was being general about his thoughts and feelings and maybe that's where it should have stayed until or unless he shifted it. And, of course, his own sensitivities to questioning – and this links back to his relationship with his mother – just made it even more difficult for him.'

'So it left you uncomfortable.'

'And that's OK, I mean, you know, we've talked about this before, but I was left wondering whether I really had responded in an unhelpful way, that while it had helped bring clarity to Peter about his sensitivity and how his childhood experiences have affected him, I did push him.'

'I'm struck by a thought here because when a therapist has a sense of pushing a client there are two elements to this. The therapist is pushing the client away from a particular focus – and that may be the key. But he is also pushing the client towards an experience – which may also be the primary factor. And it can, of course, be a bit of both. Do you sense that the significance was around what he was pushed away from, or pushed towards?'

Michael stopped to think. He hadn't really thought of it quite like that. He'd focused in his own processing more on what he had pushed Peter towards and the effect that had had. Of course, at the time, he didn't know it would provoke the reaction that it did. At least, he was not aware of this. In the moment he had thought he was being helpful, trying to enable Peter to get clarity by helping him to personalise the meaning of love in terms of his own experience. But he had pushed him away from the more general exploration. 'I need to think about this and try and recall what he was saying before my response.' He sat thinking back. Peter had been talking of his feelings for Melanie, and they had been very touching and tender, he remembered that. Then there was something about, yes, feeling embarrassed. He started to speak again. 'Yes, he spoke very touchingly about his feelings for Melanie, and wondering if what he was experiencing was love. Then I said something because it seemed like he was maybe embarrassed and he sort of confirmed it but also said it was good talking to me, that his mother wouldn't have been interested. And then I think I asked the direct question about what love meant to him, and then the reaction.'

'So, Peter had said that he was talking about something that was very important to him, embarrassed a bit by it, something he couldn't talk to his mother about – presumably she would have questioned him about it?'

'Yes, that's it, she would have done, but he was telling me and maybe within himself was feeling safe enough to do that, feeling he wouldn't get that kind of questioning. Yes, oh yes, this makes a lot of sense. Maybe he had let his guard down, so to speak, feeling more able to take the risk in spite of that sensed embarrassment, and then he gets a question which I don't think on the face of it was particularly probing, but it had the effect of, well, maybe provoking a reaction to protect himself.'

'You mean he closed down in some way?'

'I think a lot of things happened. I think he was shocked, I guess somewhere part of him was listening out for a question, to be maybe interrogated as he had received so much of that in the past, and it is a sensitive area for him to talk about, and it does require him to trust me. But my response was just too close to the kind of reaction he was used to. I mean, I thought I said it fairly gently, but it was still a question and it is that questioning tone that seems to have been the factor.' Michael paused for a moment. He suddenly felt very sorry for Peter. 'Poor guy. Takes a risk of being open about something so precious to him, something he feels he has no one else to share with, and I give him a question that set up a reaction in him that made it difficult for him to continue on that theme. I hadn't expected the reaction. And I don't think I was trying to take him away from his focus. I mean, I was by making it specific to him, but I wasn't feeling that I wanted him to get away from generalising because I was uncomfortable. Actually, I think it is a fascinating topic – trying to unravel the mystery of love – what it is, where it comes from, how we respond to it, what it means to us. I think my question was an innocent one.'

'Mhmm, but it happened around a really sensitive topic with a client feeling, perhaps, more vulnerable than you had imagined?'

'Yes, I think I had slipped up on that. And I was aware of being conscious of trying to avoid too many questions after that interaction.'

'Like you were getting a clear signal, "don't ask questions?".'

'Something like that. Or maybe it's more that the question was linked to such a sensitive area, and to a part of Peter that is developing and is still tender and needing protection?'

'That how it feels?'

'I think so. I mean, having talked one week about not feeling loved and wanting to understand why his mother hadn't loved him, to then talking about his feelings for his girlfriend and wondering what love means from the angle of being the one who is doing the loving. It's all about giving and receiving, but he didn't feel he ever received and he is struggling to know if what he is now receiving – or giving – is love. He hasn't got anything in his background he feels he can reliably measure it against. And then I try to get him to be specific and it's all too much.'

'Overloads, too uncomfortable, too close to the edge.'

'Very much so. And the session then continued but it wasn't "easy", if you know what I mean. Didn't really flow. Lots of silences. But no, then it did settle down, and he was talking about needing to get away from home, yes, that's it, not feeling able to breathe. Of being scared, as well, of losing what he has with Melanie. He talked a lot about wanting to break free, not just from home, but from himself. How did he word it? Something like "how do I break free from the me that life has made me become?", or something like that. Can't remember exactly. But he really does want to break free and I think he's increasingly aware that it isn't just about outer change, moving on in that way, it's about inner change. At the end a quote came to mind, about needing to be the change we want to see in the world, and he applied that to himself in terms of recognising that he needed to be the change he wanted to see in himself, and how he needed to take responsibility. And control. No, no, control came up in the next session. Oh yes, I have to tell you about that.'

'OK, before that, let me just see if I have the themes right here. Not feeling he was loved, confused as to what love is, scared of losing the love he has with Melanie, wanting to break free of who he is, vulnerability to questions, to not feeling heard.'

'Yes, and feeling angry and frustrated about how he is.'

'I'm thinking about the enormous scope here for Peter to have constructed within his structure of self a range of configurations.'

'Yes, that thought had struck me, too. It's not that he has necessarily identified anything specifically although there are key identities that he has built sets of feelings, thoughts and behaviours around, he has to have done.'

'Would it help to explore this?' Suzy felt that sometimes this could be helpful although she was always mindful of not wanting to construct something that may not be reflective of what the client's inner world was really like. But sometimes there could be so much, so many strands to a particular client that to try and get some image of it broken down could be helpful.

'Well, we have an angry and frustrated element, feeling not listened to, that his views are dismissed. And I can imagine there is a frustration of wanting to be heard, to make a point, to win an argument. There is that part of him that will have been modelled on his father, going invisible, or getting away, ignoring what was happening, maybe looking the other way. That seems to be with how he dealt with her.'

'OK, what else?'

'The part that wants freedom, that wants to live but maybe doesn't quite know how to. I guess this is linked to the idea of his wanting independence, to stand as a man in control of his own life and destiny.'

'You said control came up in the next session, but let's come back to that.'

'OK, but that's an important area I think. There's also the sense of feeling unlovable and of not being valued. So, wanting control but a life of being controlled, wanting freedom but a life of feeling, well, not having that freedom, not being able to affirm himself as a man. Impotence came up in the last session as well. Hm, could have maybe phrased that better.'

Suzy smiled. She let it go, didn't want to divert the focus. 'So, OK, we've got a lot of areas here, powerful aspects of Peter's structure of self that he is struggling with. Being pulled between the different sets of feelings, leaving him feeling, what, impotent to achieve change? And what about you? How is all this leaving you feeling, given you said at the start you needed to talk things through to achieve clarity and to be accurately responsive to him?' Suzy felt they had identified a number of parts of Peter, but what of Michael? How was he responding to the client?

'A bit jumbled, I guess. Lots of elements here and a client feeling stuck with them, and at the same time he does feel he has a direction to work towards. The last session we had was very significant. Brought a lot out. Well, actually, the session was simply making sense of things that had already happened.' Michael went on to describe the last session and the role that attending *Phantom of the Opera* had had on Peter and the connectedness they had experienced together during that session.

'So, that really was a powerful experience, and as you say, seems to have been extremely timely for Peter.'

'I think so. I think what was important was that he went through his own process of making connections within himself and making sense of things. It was his journey and he was, if you like, in control? He made the links with the phantom, with his past. He saw how affected he was, and how he wanted to free himself from that, and how important his love for Melanie is in this process. I don't mean he's using her, but it's how it is. They've met at a time when he needed to meet her, and maybe for her to meet him, given the role model she had from her father of what men are like. Peter's perhaps as different to her father as she is to Peter's mother.' He stopped. 'Hadn't quite put that together before now, but it's true, isn't it? They're both finding out about relating to someone of the opposite sex who is very different from their parental experience. And yet there is the similarity because for Peter, his mother took the power, the authoritarian role. So he experienced it but from the other gender.' He shook his head. 'I can see them in couple therapy at some point, although, who knows, maybe they will find ways of disentangling the conditioning themselves. Love's a powerful healer.'

'I have this image of them really holding on to each other, of just how important their relationship is in Peter's process, but in hers as well. It's kind of good that Peter doesn't just have you, that he has a female to explore things with, express himself with. He's got to learn new ways of being as an adult, as a man. But we're talking about him, and I'm aware that this keeps happening. What about you? How are you in all of this? I feel like while Peter is present here, I'm losing you. And I wonder what that's about and whether that has a meaning specific to your work with Peter.'

'Where am I? Well, I do feel for Peter. And what I was saying about that last session, that moment of connection with him – well, it was more than a moment. That was powerful. I really do feel for the guy, and really have a sense that he can move on. He wants to and he has someone, and that's great. I hope it works out for them, I mean, not that it has to be long term, but whatever happens, what they have proves fulfilling and satisfying to them both. So I do feel for him. I do feel I can listen to him. He has confirmed that. He is risking areas of himself with me. And we can only go at his pace with that. In a way it feels like he has presented so much material and in a way it is really still early days in the process. I can imagine – if he wants to – that we could be working together for quite some time. It just depends. If he does move out and in with Melanie, who knows what that will throw up, and whether he'll want to continue to work with me. Or whether they choose something for themselves as a couple. And his mother. He hasn't talked a lot about specifics recently. She's like a kind of ever-present presence that is sometimes in the foreground but generally in the background.'

'How do you feel towards her?'

Michael smiled. 'I don't know. Part of me is angry and wants to tell her to back off and let her son get on with his life, and that feels punitive towards her and rescuing towards him. Part of me, though, wants to understand her. Why was she as she was – and is? What is she getting out of this relationship? Is she stuck in some way, and what caused that stuckness? I'm sure something significant happened to her in the past, or maybe her upbringing, I don't know. But I wish they could talk. I just have this sense – and maybe this is the optimist in me – but somehow, somewhere, there can be a meeting between them. I go back in my mind to that experience Peter had as a child, when he wanted that glass of water. The reaction was too strong. Something was already going on, but maybe it worsened from that point. I don't know. Part of me feels angry towards her, but there is a part of me that wants to feel compassionate but can't find ... no, doesn't have anything to hang that compassion on. I just wish they could find some way of sitting down and talking it out.'

'You sound very passionate about that, Michael, you really believe that could happen?'

'I don't know. I like to think so. If he never was loved, wanted, valued, there had to be a reason. Why did she turn against him? Why? I mean, he wasn't the oldest so it couldn't have been that she'd had to marry his father who maybe she didn't want. I don't know. Fruitless speculating. But there has to be something.'

'You sound frustrated and I'm aware you mentioned anger as well, similar feelings to Peter.'

'Yes, well, I can imagine what it must be like. It wasn't my experience, and yes, maybe I have to watch feeling angry and frustrated on his behalf. And yet I also have to own the presence of those feelings. Talking about his mother now does help me to soften but it is frustrating as well. But it's the long haul. Isn't it? I can't make anything happen. Not my role, and certainly not my way of working. Go with it. Things are happening for Peter. Experiences are mounting up in his life, pushing him, forcing him to look at himself, his world, his choices, his behaviours. Actually, the impact of *Phantom of the Opera* felt really good. It's like life is taking him on a journey and I often think that we lose sight of that. We can think that therapy is the central factor in people changing, growing, doing what they do, but actually it's a part of a greater process. An important part, but just a part. And I believe as therapists we have to work in such a way that we collaborate with the life process. I don't just mean the actualising tendency, but the events, experiences, occurrences that arise in our clients' lives. I have to work with the bigger picture with Peter but also be mindful and attentive to the specifics. And that's challenging, but exciting as well.'

'You look suddenly as though you've been given a gift.' Suzy wasn't quite sure why she said it, but it sort of seemed to reflect what she was feeling. 'There's a kind of youthful enthusiasm in the way you are speaking.'

'Peter is a gift. Yes. He's what I need. I've got my life process too. And I really value working with him. It fills me with enthusiasm. I don't know what will happen next and that is exciting. Whenever I talk to you I always seem to gain enthusiasm. Not that I come through the door without it, but I do leave with it. So thanks for that.'

'Thanks for that. Look, we really have ranged across all kinds of things here with regard to Peter and your work with him. It is complex. There is a lot going on for him that is impacting on you. You talked about wanting to feel clear. Talking about him as we have, and about your reactions and feelings, has it helped?'

'Yes, it has. I do feel clearer. It is complex and jumbled and in a way our process here has paralleled that I think. But having the space to let the jumble out has somehow helped to clear things. And I know I need to stay with Peter, at his pace, and really offer him that warm and accepting space for him to take the risks he needs to take, to bring the experiences that he is having, the confusions, the questions, the struggles and the joys.' Michael smiled. 'Yes, and the joys. And I hope that he can have more of those. He knows he can. He knows what feels good in his life at the moment and it is forcing him to confront patterns from his past. His need to love, to be loved, is driving him onwards.'

The supervision session moved on to a discussion about another of Michael's clients. At the end of the session, as Michael left, he found himself thinking once more about Peter and his struggle to love, to understand the meaning of love. It was a theme he'd pondered on himself, and had had his own experiences. He had known what it was like to love and feel loved, and he knew how incredibly powerful the experience was, how beautiful and exquisite it could be. The simple fact of knowing you are loved, and feeling that love. In the world today, particularly the 'developed' world with all its hype and intensity, where was the space, the time, for love to flourish? And how can you be open to love when it had never been offered to you, a childhood bereft of that sense of feeling wanted?

For some, it is a case that the meaning of love is distorted – people who are sexually abused but made to feel special. Made to feel that that is what love is about who then perpetuate this themselves, or seek relationships that ensure they remain targets of abuse. But for Peter, it was different. He was unsure whether he had felt love and he really was not sure what it was. And now he was learning, and fast, through his relationship with Melanie. What would happen with his relationship with his mother? There had to be a reason why things had been as they were. There had to be. But he did not have an answer.

CHAPTER 8

Counselling session 11: a night in the cells, time to move on

10 November

The calmness had stayed with Peter for a while after the last session. He felt strangely detached from things at home, doing what he wanted, when he wanted. He spent more time with Melanie, more nights with her. His mother, at the end of the week, made the suggestion that perhaps he should bring 'this Melanie' round to meet her on the Sunday. Peter had said no, not if that was her attitude. They'd actually made other plans anyway and Peter was reluctant to change those, particularly given that he didn't think his mother was going to make her very welcome. It didn't help the atmosphere at home when he said no, and explained why. He got a torrent of verbal abuse from his mother and it was at that point that something snapped in Peter. He'd had enough. An invisible line had been crossed.

Peter sat in the waiting area; he was a few minutes early. He'd been given a coffee and was thumbing through a magazine. There happened to be an article in one of them that looked at how adults who experienced disruption, chaos and uncertainty in childhood were left feeling and behaving as adults. He read some of the characteristics and realised that they very much described his mother and, to a certain degree as well, himself. It left him wondering about her past. He knew so little about her early life. Her parents had died early and she'd been brought up by foster parents. He'd known them as an aunt and uncle: auntie Rose and uncle Derek. But he'd only met them a couple of times, years ago as a child. He hadn't any clear memory of them, and his mother never spoke of them. He heard Michael calling his name and it brought him out of his thoughts.

'How are things?'

'Not too bad really. Been a bit of a week.' As he spoke, Peter was still aware that he had the article in his head, and wasn't really focused on what he was saying.

'Mhmm. Bit of a week?' Michael allowed his curiosity to be present in his tone of voice and waited to see if Peter wanted to say more about it.

'Oh, well, usual stuff, and a big blow up with my mother.'

'Bigger than usual?'

Peter nodded. 'Yeah, really big. I snapped. I mean, I've been frustrated and irritated for some while, and yes, I get angry, but this time she just went too far.' He explained how his mother had suggested that he bring Melanie over, 'but it was the way she said "this Melanie". It was quite clear she didn't really want to meet her, not with any warmth anyway. Anyway, I said "no", not if she was going to take that attitude. And then, well, it just escalated into a stand-up argument – well, more of a slanging match really. I think a lot of my frustration over the years got unleashed. And, well, she said some really awful things as well, told me how she'd always done her best for me, how she still put up with me, gave me a home. I told her how crap her best had been, and, well, that I'd never felt loved or cared for and I was only at home out of a sense of duty. And, well, you can imagine, all kinds of things got said and it really got out of control. Anyway, I left, I was seething and in fact I actually wasn't sure that I trusted myself. I did get to the point of feeling I wanted to lash out at her, and that really isn't me. So I went out. Didn't know where to go. Melanie was having an evening with girlfriends – this was the Friday – and I ended up going for a walk, and finally wound up in a local pub, and got drunk. Not something I generally do, but that's what happened. Staggered back later in the evening to find the door locked and I couldn't get in. Tried to wake her up, ringing the bell, threw stones at her window. Anyway, someone must have called the police, they arrived and I was taken away. Spent the night in the cells, sobering up. They're not pressing charges, fortunately. I realised then that that was it, I wasn't going to be able to live there any more.' He paused for moment before continuing. Michael did not interrupt, allowing the story to unfold.

'Next morning I went round to Melanie's and explained the situation and, well, I've organised a small flat, well, more of a bedsit really, where I'm going to move in to later in the week. And I'm currently staying with Melanie temporarily. The people she shares the house with are OK, so long as it is temporary, and I've made it clear that it is. So, that's where I'm at. Can't believe it really. Everything happened so quickly, but I guess I needed this to make it happen. It's really forced the issue.'

Michael listened carefully to what Peter was saying. He wondered whether he had had further contact with his mother. But he knew that was his curiosity and he set it aside.

'So, bit of a week is a bit of an understatement. You've moved out and it's been an intense time all round.'

'I'm really sorry that things have happened the way that they have, but maybe they had to. I don't know. I've spoken to my mother, and she first of all just started at me again, and I found that difficult and ended up putting the phone down on her. That wasn't something I would have expected to have done, but it just set me off. I could feel myself reacting, I could feel the anger inside myself again building up. I just didn't want to hear her.'

'Mhmm, had enough, didn't want to hear her going on at you.'

'No.' He shook his head. 'So, now, well, we'll have to see. I went back round to get some clothes. She was out, fortunately. Left a note to say she could call me on my mobile. Told her I'd be back to sort out my stuff another time, and that was that.'

Michael nodded, aware that he was hearing the story and, yes, the anger was there but he sensed the sadness as well.

'Hmm. Must leave you with a lot of different thoughts and feelings.'

Peter took a deep breath. Yes, he thought to himself, yes. He swallowed. 'I didn't want it to be like this, but I know I can't talk to her, not the way I feel at the moment. But it does leave me feeling sorry that it has happened. I . . .' He stopped, not sure what to say next. He hadn't wanted it to be like this. It wasn't what he had planned or expected. He hadn't been sure how he would leave, though he knew he had to. But he hadn't wanted all this anger and bitterness. And his mind wandered back to the article he'd been reading in the waiting area. He'd forgotten about it as he had been talking.

'Just before I came in, I was reading an article out there in a magazine, about how chaos in childhood affects you as an adult, and I saw my mother. And it left me wondering what kind of experience she had, and what effect all this is having on her. And I wonder if I'm just being selfish here, and whether I should try and, oh I don't know, make peace somehow, and yet I also know part of me doesn't want to.'

'Mhmm. Part of you wants to make peace with your mother and feels you're being selfish, and another part isn't so sure about that.'

'I guess, well, I guess I have to make peace eventually, and maybe sooner is better than later. But I don't know. I feel so reactive at the moment. And I'm so glad I have somewhere to be at the moment. When the police arrived, well, that was a real shock. Never had a night in the cells, but it gave me time to think – although my thoughts probably weren't too sharp. I hadn't drunk much, I guess I was more angry and frustrated than drunk, but I had had a few. And that just isn't me. But I didn't know what to do or where to go. I had thought of going round to one of the guys from work, who I get on with quite well. But I wasn't sure exactly where he lived so there wasn't much point in that. So that's when I started making more noise to try to wake her up, and then, well, you know the rest.'

'Must have been quite a shock?'

'It is now I look back. I guess, at the time, I wasn't thinking too clearly. So, yes, a shock but . . . And sitting in that cell, I mean, it wasn't that I was behind bars as such, but my thoughts went back to the phantom, being exhibited in a cage. Not that I was being exhibited, but I guess I'd made an exhibition of myself and had ended up locked up because of it. Thinking about that made me more determined to make a new life for myself. So, I do see it as positive, I know I have to move on, and it is happening. But I'm not sure how I'm going to handle the fall-out, as it were.'

'The fall-out?'

'My mother.'

Michael nodded. 'Yeah, how to handle her reaction.'

Peter sat for a moment thinking. He hadn't any answers. He didn't know what to say, and it didn't feel like the time to try and say it. Words had been said between them and they still hurt. And he wasn't prepared to feel hurt again.

'I need a break from her. No wonder Barry and Lucy got away. Wish I had.'

'You wish you'd got away sooner?'

'Yeah, but, you know, like I said, my dad's death and everything, felt I had to stay around. But that's in the past now. I can't use that as a reason any more. I mean, that's not healthy. I . . . I don't know, maybe I should go and visit Barry, go and meet him, take Melanie. We're in touch, though I think he looks down on me as well, but not like mother did. But maybe, yeah, maybe I need to go and see him, put him in the picture. I can just see my mother telling him her view of what has happened. Not that they have much contact, but maybe she'll call him.'

'So, visiting Barry is an option.'

'Yes, and maybe we can talk about the past. Maybe he knows something that I don't. I don't know. We've never talked about it before. And maybe we should. Well, maybe I need to. I don't know.' He paused again. 'I'm sure something happened to my mother; I can't believe she is naturally how she is.'

'It seems really important for you to believe that.'

Peter nodded. 'Yes, the thought that she might, well, naturally be this way. So much venom sometimes. Like poison. As though she's trying to spit it out, but does so by spitting it at others.'

'That's how it feels, spitting out poison, and you were a target.'

'I need to speak to Barry. I'm going to see if I can arrange to go up there. Can't be this week, too much to do, but maybe the following weekend. I'll give him a ring one evening, tell him what's happened. I want someone in my family to meet Melanie as well, I mean, I feel so good about being with her, you know, I want to kind of show her off, and, yeah, be a couple. I've got to do this. It's important to me.'

Michael was unsure precisely what it was that was important and he sought to clarify this. 'Important for you to be as a couple, or for her, or you together, to be seen, known by your family?'

'Just want to find some normality, you know, be able to be with my family with Melanie. Just do a normal thing. I can't do it at home, well, it's not my home now. But just, I don't know . . .' He took a deep breath and sighed. 'I just want to get on with my life with Melanie and do normal things and, yes, I want our relationship to be accepted in some way by my family.'

'Mhmm, your relationship with Melanie, to feel that it is accepted by family.'

'And as you say that back to me, my reaction is, "why?". Why is it so important? And yet it is, and I guess, well, I guess that's to do with me and my not feeling wanted. Maybe I'm . . . Shit!' He paused and tightened his lips as the uncomfortable thought struck him. 'Maybe I'm hoping that through Melanie I'll feel wanted.' Another deep breath and a long sigh. 'No, that's not how it is. I hadn't been thinking about bringing Melanie home, it all came about because of what my mother said. Up till then, we were just getting on with our lives. I knew somewhere along the line she would have to meet mother, but I guess I was putting that away, not really wanting to focus too much on that.'

Michael responded, 'So, you weren't feeling an urge to introduce Melanie to your family, but the issue got forced by your mother's invitation.'

'If that's what it was. Yes.' He paused while he thought again. 'There has to be something wrong with her, Michael. I don't know what, but I don't understand why she has been the way that she has for so many years. She's alienated Lucy and Barry, and now me. Why did she hate us?'

'Powerful question – why did she hate you all?'

'Maybe hate's too strong a word for it, but she didn't want us, well, no, she wanted us to do things for her, but . . . oh, I don't know, the questions give me a headache and in a way I'm fed up with asking them. But I can't stop. It's like a tape going round and round in my head sometimes. And I can't answer it. And I can't stop it. "Why me? Why us? Why? Why? Why?" ' Peter shook his head while taking a breath and rubbing his face with his hands. 'I'm tired of it all, Michael, I'm so tired of it all. I need to move on, make a fresh start, create a new life.'

'All the "whys?" remain unanswered, you're tired of the questions, you know you have to move on to a new life.'

Peter nodded. It was good to hear back those words. Yes, he was fed up with the questions and, yes, he had to make a new start. He had to. Hearing the words helped him confirm to himself the reality of what he wanted.

'Maybe I'll find out one day, and maybe it'll be when the time is right. Hell, things have happened to me these last few weeks that I wasn't anticipating. I mean, coming here, meeting up with Melanie, and now moving out and moving on. I mean, if I'd known that all this was going to happen – not to mention the night in the cells – I wouldn't have believed it.'

'So there's an element of it all being unbelievable, and yet it's happening.'

'And I want to ask, "what next?", and I don't know that I want an answer!'

Michael smiled; yes, he thought, if we knew ahead what was going to happen, who knows what we would do? 'So, you want to take things as they come rather than know what lies ahead?'

'Very much so, although I also want to know that things will be OK. I mean, I guess I want to know the future, but only to be reassured that all will be OK?'

'So if it's a good future, you want to know. If it's a bad future . . .'

'. . . then I don't want to know.' Peter shook his head. 'Crazy stuff. Anyway, my priority now is to get myself moved into this small flat – and it is small, but at least it will be my space and I'm kind of looking forward to that. Rent's not too bad, and, well, hopefully it won't be too long before Melanie and I can organise something for ourselves. That's the plan. We don't want to rush into it – we talked about renting together now, but decided it would be too rushed, we want to find the right place. So we'll take our time.'

'Mhmm, makes sense, take your time, and I guess for me what I sense is something about taking control.'

'Hmm, yes, you're right. Yes, it is about that, isn't it? Taking control. Making decisions that we want to make. And that feels good.' He stopped again as uncomfortable feelings surfaced once more. 'But . . . I feel responsible for my mother as well, and how she must be feeling. And do I have the right to be like this, I mean, I feel like I'm being selfish.'

'That's how it feels, like you are being selfish?' Michael was tempted to emphasise the 'you' but that would have been directive and the result of his own reaction which was that Peter had nothing to feel selfish about, that he'd gone more than the extra mile to be with his mother, and that he'd reached that point of having to move on.

'That was something from childhood. Always being told not to be selfish, always think of others. Always share what we had with each other. And yet always, "put family first", yes, I'd forgotten that, always "blood thicker than water". It was so constraining, looking back, so inward looking. I guess it's all tied in with her childhood – losing her parents and being with uncle Derek and auntie Rose, maybe she wanted to feel part of a family, maybe she didn't feel that, and was desperate somehow to, I don't know. Maybe she just didn't know about how to be in a family. And then, I don't know, I'm back thinking about that incident when I was three with the glass of water, and the man with my mother. Who was he? So many questions. They just keep going round and round, more so since I've been coming here. Guess I'm more aware of them, plus I've got more in touch with some of my past.'

Michael nodded. Yes, he thought, therapy so often contributed to change. It wasn't that it caused it necessarily, though often it did. But sometimes therapy was simply another piece in the jigsaw of change. Yes, he could understand the mixed feeling that Peter had. Wondering, as well, what may have been in his mother's past. He was struck by the role of loss in Peter's mother's life. Lost her parents, her husband, two children moved away as soon as they could, and now Peter moving out. Loss seemed to be a key factor. He had long been aware of how people seemed to experience the thing they feared most. And yet his mother's behaviour hadn't seemed to be that which would hold people in relationship with her, and that felt like a contradiction. These thoughts were running in the background as Michael responded to what Peter had been saying.

'Yes, so many questions unanswered, not knowing what your mother's childhood was like, and why "blood is thicker than water" was somehow so important.'

Peter just knew he had no answers, but he did want to find out. The more he thought about it, the more he knew he wanted to reach out to her, as he had done throughout his life, but whereas in the past it was in order to feel loved, now it was different. He wanted to understand her. He also felt irritated and angry as well, but there was a sense of wanting to help, if that was possible. But he also knew now wasn't perhaps the time.

'There has to be a reason. Maybe I'll understand one day. Maybe. It's sad to have come to this, but maybe it was inevitable. And maybe, in the long run, well, maybe something will happen to help me understand her. At the moment, though, I know I'm too angry, too much still bottled up inside me, to really listen to her.'

Michael could hear the sadness in Peter's voice. Yes, he was angry, but sad as well. 'I hear the anger, and I hear the sadness in your voice as well.'

'I've said it before, I can't breathe when I'm with her, I feel suffocated, but I hadn't fully appreciated how much until now, at least, the last few weeks. Melanie has opened me up to a whole new world, a new part of myself, and I have to stay with that.'

His voice still sounded very sad to Michael. 'Something new and exciting, allowing you to breathe.' He did not comment on the sadness. He'd mentioned it in his previous response and Peter had chosen not to pick it up. He needed to stay with the part of Peter's inner world that he wanted to communicate. 'You have to stay with it, yes?'

'Yes, I have to.' He paused, being aware of how just how important it was. 'Yes, I *have* to.'

'That important. So important.' Michael, rather than getting into what felt like verbal table-tennis of just batting the same words back and forward, switched to emphasising the importance which, though it is not a word that was used, was present in the tone and meaning of what was being said.

'I'm at a crossroads, and I think, well, maybe I've chosen the route I'm taking. I can't remember if I spoke to you about a sense of being at a kind of fork in the road, maybe I was talking to Melanie, but I've made a choice, I can't look back.' He went quiet, suddenly aware of a feeling of uncertainty. He pushed it away, didn't want to feel it. 'No, can't look back.'

Michael had sensed the momentary hesitation. 'Can't look back and yet there sounds like there's a touch of hesitancy.'

Peter had been maintaining eye contact until he heard Michael's comment, and he instinctively found himself looking down. 'Yes, there is, it's a big step. I haven't been on my own like this before. I mean, OK, I'm with Melanie at the moment, but actually living on my own, that's new. I guess I'm feeling very aware of how big this change is.' He felt his arms heavy and almost numb, and a kind of coldness in the pit of his stomach. It didn't feel good. He blew out a deep breath. 'I hope it's going to work out.' He was immediately struck by a fear of what would happen if he lost Melanie, what if something didn't work out, and then he really was on his own. It wasn't a new thought, but one that he had kept well away from his day-to-day awareness. But now it was very present.

The silence struck Michael quite acutely, and the way that Peter had said that he hoped it would work out. Somehow, his certainty didn't seem quite so strong in the way that he had spoken. It seemed to Michael that a very important phase of the session had arrived. Peter was feeling vulnerable, perhaps, uncertain, unsure. He had to have these feelings somewhere inside him, the change he was making was so big. And happening so fast. Maybe he hadn't really had time to process it, or maybe the implications were only now beginning to catch up with him.

'Sounds like it has to work out.'

'The thought of it not, of something going wrong with Melanie . . .' He blew out his breath again, clearly lost in his own thoughts. Peter was shaking his head. 'The thought of being on my own like that just leaves me feeling cold, utterly, utterly cold. And empty. And yet full, full of numbness. Sounds crazy, but yes, that's how it feels.' He felt himself feeling emotional, his throat was burning, there was a lump in his throat and his eyes were feeling very moist. He took a deep breath, held it for a moment before letting it back out slowly. He was staring at the wall to the right of Michael. But he wasn't seeing it. He was so full of . . . It seemed like he had so many feelings and yet he couldn't feel them. It was a weird sensation. He thought of Melanie; he knew he had so much love for her, and yet, in the moment, he couldn't feel it. He thought of his mother; he couldn't feel his anger. He sat, staring, feeling but not feeling, looking but not looking, thinking but not thinking.

He heard Michael speaking. 'Feeling numb. Cold, empty and full of numbness.'

Peter closed his eyes. He was not in a comfortable place. His head felt suddenly full, like it wanted to burst; his eyes felt gritty. He tried to stifle a yawn, but couldn't. He suddenly felt overwhelmingly tired. He knew the session was about to finish. He deliberately closed his eyes, scrunching them up a little, and promptly yawned again. His back had stiffened. He moved to release it.

'I'm in a very different place to last week. I feel a bit spaced out, and it's not a comfortable feeling.'

'Do you need to sit a little longer, get your bearings?'

'I'll be OK. Just a bit more sensitive to the enormity of it all. I'll be OK. It's going to be one hell of a week this one. Hell of a week. Perhaps the most important week of my life. Perhaps.'

'Hmm. Moving on. Yes.' Michael wasn't sure what to say in all honesty. Yes, it was going to be an important week and he had not got the faintest idea how Peter would react. How do you anticipate your reactions when you know you are about to do something that is new to you? How would he react to being on his own? How would his mother react once he removed his stuff from the house, assuming he had space to take it all. It was going to be a testing time. But at least he had Melanie, someone who he clearly cared deeply about. He kind of wanted to meet her, wondered what she was like. He put the thought aside.

They confirmed the time for the next appointment as Peter was getting up and putting on his coat. 'Thanks, again. I'm sure I'll have a lot to talk about next time. I know what I have to do, but I guess I'm maybe a little more aware now that there is a hesitancy in me, but I have to push on regardless. I'll see you next week.'

'OK. You take care of yourself, and I'll see you next week.'

Michael had returned to the counselling room, aware that he was engaging with Peter at such a crucial and perhaps, as he had said, at a pivotal time in his life. He was moving on. The situation had been forced on him. Was he psychologically prepared? What would have enabled him to be if he wasn't? Life isn't like that. Didn't John Lennon say something along the lines that life is what happens to you when you are busy planning your next step? He knew that wasn't the quote, but he felt it captured the flavour of it. Life was happening to Peter. And no doubt the process was going to run for a while.

Counselling session 12: the truth revealed, Peter is left confused

17 November

'Well, I've moved out. Feels strange but good, but that's not all that has happened.'

'What else?' Michael could feel that there was more that Peter wanted/needed to say.

'Well, I was with my mother sorting out my stuff, what to take, you know. And, well, she started to try and make me feel guilty about leaving her. Kept asking me "why?". She told me that she hadn't heard me the night the police took me away, said she'd taken some sleeping tablets. I don't know whether that's true. Anyway, she kept saying that I should stay with her, that she didn't understand why I had to go.' He paused.

'So the question of "why?" was what concerned her?'

'Yes. Anyway, she kept on and, well, eventually I had to say something. I mean, I've been more fired up recently, you know, more determined and, well, I just had to say something. So I did.' He paused again.

Michael waited, giving time for Peter to say what he had to say in his own way and at his own pace.

'I asked her to sit down, which she did, and I sat down opposite her, and I asked her, very simply, and very directly, "Why do I experience you as having never loved or wanted me?" I carefully worded the question. I'd been thinking about it for a while since the last session. I kind of wanted to have a wording that felt right should the occasion arise.'

'Sounds like a pretty clear and direct question to me.' Michael was struck by the clarity; it really did convey what Peter wanted to know and yet without sounding blaming or being designed to antagonise. He'd have been pleased to have come up with such wording himself.

'She denied it, of course, said I was being silly. But I was strong. I said, "Look, mother, I know what I have felt over the years. I need to understand why. If you won't answer me, then I have to accept that, and I am sorry because I want to understand." She shook her head in response and said nothing, looking away from me. Then she turned to me and said, "It's you seeing that counsellor, putting weird ideas in your head. They're just busybodies, getting into other people's lives. Told you it would do you no good." I replied by saying that it had done me a lot of good, that it had helped me make sense of a number of things but I still had questions that I could not answer, one of which was why she was always critical and rejecting of me. "What had I done?" She still refused to say anything.'

Michael listened attentively; there was nothing for him to say. Peter needed to relate the details of what had happened. They would deal with the effect on him later if necessary.

'So I said, "OK, but I am moving out, I need to get a life for myself, I need my independence." ' Peter was quite calm as he spoke, and he had felt quite calm at the time as well. He had been really pleased that he had spoken as he had and that he had not lost it.

'So you made it very clear and stayed very firm?'

'I did. It wasn't easy. I was feeling quite emotional. Been in that house for a long while, well, since before my father died, so it has a lot of memories. I told her this, told her it wasn't easy for me either, but it had to happen sooner or later, and that it was happening now. I told her that I planned to spend more time with Melanie and that we were looking towards moving in somewhere together, but that we weren't rushing into it.'

Michael could hear the emotion in Peter's voice. 'You really did put her in the picture, and I can hear from your voice how much emotion you have in all of this.'

'Yes, well, not surprising really. Anyway, she still refused to see anything so I got up and carried on with packing, you know.'

Peter took a deep breath. This was the easy bit. He was very much there, back in the house with her. 'Anyway, she went away, I don't know where, but I went on with what I was doing. I don't know how much later it was, but she came up with a mug of tea for me, and sat herself down. She looked like she had been crying. She was very quiet. Not seen her like that, well, not since dad died.'

Michael nodded. The room felt very quiet. He didn't feel there was anything for him to say. He continued to listen to what Peter was saying, maintaining eye contact – which was quite spontaneous.

'She said that she had something to show me. She had a photo, an old black and white photo, of a man in army clothes.' Peter went silent. 'I recognised him immediately, but didn't say anything. He was the man who had been in bed with her that night I wanted a glass of water. But I didn't want to say anything. I wanted to hear what she had to say. Anyway, it seems that he was someone she had met at a dance, and they had fallen in love, but her father thought him "unsuitable". He was a military man, with contacts, and it seems that he must have said something to get this chap posted overseas. He was away for quite some time and, well, it seems that she then met my father and, well, seems like one night they had got drunk and, well, one thing led to another and she ended up pregnant. She had to marry my father and while there was some affection, her heart was still with this other chap – his name was Jimmy. He was from Aberdeen originally though his family had moved south and they lived nearby. Anyway, my mother had Barry and then Lucy, but she kept in touch with Jimmy. They'd meet up occasionally. Then I came along when both Barry and Lucy had started school, and she had planned to find ways of being with Jimmy, who was self-employed, during the day when they were at school. But my arrival made that difficult.'

'So you made it difficult to be with Jimmy, who she really loved?'

Peter was nodding. 'Then it seems that my father started a new job that involved him travelling and being away sometimes. Not often, but occasionally, and my mother would arrange to meet Jimmy and, well, sometimes he'd come over and stay the night with her.'

'And you saw him on one of those nights?'

Peter nodded. 'Apparently that was the last time that she saw him. Seems that somehow what happened that night made him stay away. Though I think my father changed his job around then and so maybe that also had something to do with it. But, it all ended. And it seems that I was blamed. I'd already stopped their plans by being born, and then appearing in the bedroom that night, well, for whatever reason, Jimmy didn't come back again.'

'I don't know what to say, Peter, I'm touched by what I've heard but I am wondering how it has left you feeling?'

'I didn't know what to say. We spent a few moments in silence, and then I gave her a hug, and we cried. I guess I was left feeling quite confused still. I mean,

I had answers but somehow I felt disorientated as well. It was like I had answers but now I didn't know what to do with them?'

Michael nodded. 'Yes, you now know why, but what to do with it?'

'I don't know, I still don't know. But now so much makes sense to me. Why she didn't like any of us, but why I got the worst of it. I feel somehow lost, like I also know that she didn't really love my father, and, well, I guess he knew it. It must have been awful for him, for both of them.'

'Mhmm. So you know why you got the worst of it.'

'But . . . I mean, it's no excuse, not really. I mean, it wasn't my fault. I felt sad at the time but I've also felt angry as well since that conversation with her. Felt lots of things. Confused. Angry. Sad. Lost. I've talked to her on the phone and visited her a couple of times over the weekend, and, well, things are easier somehow, but it's going to take time to come to terms with all of this.'

Michael nodded in response. 'Yes, it is likely to take time to absorb it all.'

'So, there we are. A sudden twist to everything. Last week I was so angry and fired up. Today I feel quite subdued, very reflective and, as I say, feeling confused, though it's hard to really describe it. It's like I'm living a little bit on automatic pilot. Just going through the motions much of the time. At other times I'm OK. Been seeing Melanie and she's been really supportive. She's coming over to meet mum next weekend. I was hesitant at first when mother suggested it, but she wanted to and, well, things do seem very different now. I'm still coming to terms with it all.'

'It seems that you are finding it so hard to come to terms with it all, and it is early days, of course. You say confused and, well, I'm kind of with the word "disorientated", and I guess moving out as well in the midst of all of this has probably added to what you are experiencing.'

'Yes, although I haven't actually spent much time on my own. What with being with Melanie and visiting mum, and work, you know?

'Mhmm, not much time to be on your own at the new place.'

'And maybe that's a good thing, I don't know. But it's how it is and, well, everything has changed.'

'Yes, everything has changed.'

They both lapsed into silence.

'So, I guess mum and I will keep talking and maybe things will be OK. She's not had a go at me at all since I moved out, and I really am surprised. I'm not sure that she loves me though, even now. I think she doesn't really know who to love, or maybe how to love having felt so bitter and resentful for so long. But at least I do now, and I have Melanie to thank for that.'

'So, yes, unsure whether you will ever feel love from your mother, but the truth is out and you have Melanie in your life.'

'Yes.' Silence again. Peter was back to counting the petals on flower heads on the painting on the wall. He wasn't consciously doing it, but just found himself staring at it. She loves me, she loves me not, he thought to himself. He thought about Melanie, but he knew she loved him. Then about his mother, and, well, he didn't know, but maybe now, maybe with things out in the open, perhaps things would stay changed for the better.

'Of course, Barry and Lucy don't know.'

Michael had wondered but was surprised the way that Peter had just suddenly said it.

'So only you and your mum know, then?'

Peter nodded. 'She doesn't want me to say anything. She thinks that perhaps she will, one day, maybe, but not yet. I've agreed not to say anything but did point out that maybe it might help to heal the rifts, although there's no guarantee how they'll both react. I still think it was unfair. I can appreciate her feelings, but I was her son, we were her children. However much we may have stopped her being with the man she loved, we were her own flesh and blood . . .' He stopped. 'Blood thicker than water? Another connection. And feeling caged, like the phantom, and she was caged in a relationship she didn't want to be in with children she didn't want – at least, not with our dad. What a mess. And yet, there's no excuse for how she has been towards us. Not really. And that's what's so difficult to accept. But, well, I have to find a way to live with that and be grateful for the love I have with Melanie and hope that we can make it work. I know we haven't really known each other long, but, well, I'm hopeful. But I feel like I have a lot more work to do on myself, to really resolve the effects of my upbringing. I hope you can help.' He looked at Michael, who nodded a response.

'Yes, there's a lot to come to terms with, but human beings are good at that. And you've got a future to work towards as well as a past to come to terms with. And it will all happen in the present.'

'So, that's the situation. I want to move on still, want to get a grip on my life, but somehow I feel I need to just take my time a little, adjust gradually, maybe rebuild my relationship with my mother and hope things don't slide back into the old pattern. I don't think it will. So I hope that she can accept me as I am, and for who I am, and get on with Melanie, and if we achieve that, well, that's a start.'

'That's the goal at the moment, rebuild relationships and bring Melanie into the picture.'

The session continued. Peter was quite subdued. He wasn't feeling like saying much more. He felt he had needed to come and tell Michael what had happened. He wanted to continue with the counselling; he knew he needed it to come to terms with everything and to have someone to explore what was happening for him, and to check out anything that needed checking out. He also felt he was carrying baggage from the past, unfinished business, unresolved experiences that left him still feeling vulnerable to criticism.

Towards the end of the session Peter made the comment, 'Knowing what happened changes things and yet doesn't change them. So I have an answer. My head can tell me what happened and why. But it can't get rid of how I see myself, how I experience who I am. It can't take away what has happened, how I've been treated and what effect that has had. That's going to take time, isn't it?'

Michael had nodded. 'Yes, but we cannot be sure how long. You've made a lot of progress, Peter, in 12 sessions. A lot has happened. Some might have been anticipated, but a lot has occurred and has contributed to the process.'

Peter left, still feeling reflective. He was heading back to his flat. He was still aware of having mixed up feelings about everything but he had left the counselling reassured that that was normal and OK, and that it would settle down when the time was right. He knew deep down he was doing the right thing, but he also wanted to try and work on his relationship with his mother.

Michael sat in the counselling chair staring at the wall. He was tired, very tired. It had been a long day. He had not expected Peter to have told his mother, or for the story to have come out, but he was glad that it had. At least everyone now had a better chance of being real with each other. He hoped that Barry and Lucy would be told, and that this would afford an opportunity for the healing process to begin – or at least, at this stage, an opportunity to begin to clean out the wounds as a prerequisite to healing. Yes, he thought, clean out the wounds, the psychological and emotional wounds of family life. Sons and mothers. Mothers and sons. Just one dynamic in the heady mix of family relationships.

Points for discussion

- What are your reactions to what has been disclosed in this session?
- Have your feelings changed towards Peter and/or his mother, and what impact would that have on you as Peter's counsellor?
- What would you feel you would need to take to supervision?
- Write your own notes for this session.
- What key issues do you anticipate will need to be addressed in future counselling sessions?
- What key qualities do you think Michael offered Peter over the course of the 12 sessions?
- Evaluate Michael's overall effectiveness as a person-centred counsellor.
- Evaluate Suzy's effectiveness as a person-centred supervisor.
- What specific points will you take away from reading this book?

CHAPTER 9

Peter reflects on his experience so far

I really didn't know what to expect from counselling, and for a long while I was unsure whether it was helpful. But in the end, I realised that although it wasn't a comfortable process, it has made a huge difference. Hard to know exactly what it was that had the effect, though. I mean, feelings, memories seemed to emerge as time went on, and then the things happening in my own life seem to add more meaning to it all. It was more of a process than a specific event. To try to say that a particular experience in counselling made the difference, well, I can't point to anything. I mean, I know reliving that experience as a child asking for the drink of water, yes, that was significant. But did it cause me to change? I don't know.

In many ways it was the experiences outside of the counselling that seemed to make the difference. Perhaps I made more of them, or they made more of me. I don't know. But certainly seeing *Phantom of the Opera* had a big effect. It really did put me in touch with aspects of myself and my experience. It reinforced my need to move on, which I'd also got strongly in touch with through that song, 'Bat Out of Hell'. Yet I feel that somehow both had the impact that they had because I was seeing Michael, because I was already seeking change even though I wasn't really too sure where I was heading.

Of course, the really big change in my life was meeting Melanie and falling in love with her. I guess, though, that it only happened because I was changing, looking for something new, giving myself a chance of a new experience. She was very much at the heart of my process of change. When you think about it, I only went to see *Phantom* because I was with her. It was my mother's attitude towards her that was such a catalyst as well in my deepening realisation of my need to move out and move on. She's been there for me and I have learned to love and to be loved through her.

There was a lot of emotion released in those counselling sessions and I am sure there will be more in the future. Although I have made some big decisions in my life, I know I have to work further on myself. There are outer changes, yes, but I feel the need for more inner change, or perhaps to feel that the inner changes are more secure. So I will continue with the counselling.

As I sit thinking about the journey so far, I realise that perhaps some of the really significant moments were not about talking. The physical contact was at times unsettling and yet it also gave me something which I find hard to put into words. I felt Michael's care and I experienced a kind of reassurance when he made contact with me, and when he held me during the really difficult, emotional moments. I still don't think I ever really experienced that kind of contact as a child. I may be wrong. I know how memory can play tricks and it is easy to forget. But my sense is that this was a new experience and, as an adult man to be held by another man, that was quite challenging to me. And yet it was also very much OK as well. It began to get easier. And maybe that is also linked to my developing physical relationship with Melanie which has also helped me feel freer and more confident with physical contact. And I know that if, at the start, some-one had said to me that the most powerful experience you will have in therapy will be being physically held by another man, I'd probably have run a mile. Strange. But that's how it is.

As for my relationship with my mother, who knows? We are both on a learning curve now, perhaps I should say on our own individual learning curves. Perhaps they will converge. I hope so. I would like to genuinely feel good about her, but not simply that desperate wanting to feel good when deep down I didn't. It's been difficult for her too, but I hope we can move on. I hope that she and Melanie get along. That is important to me; however, I do know that if they do not, it won't get in the way of the relationship Melanie and I are building. My mother domi-nated my past; Melanie is very much part of my present and I hope will be in my future too. I have to work towards the future that I want, and it would be great if my mother could share that in a way that we all felt good about.

Yes, Michael listened, though at times he did make it difficult for me, particu-larly with his questions. But I'm learning to handle that. I've certainly learned to trust him more and more, and that feels really important. So, as I say, it has not been comfortable or easy, and I am amazed at how I have changed and how my life has changed over these past few months. Talking to a stranger – I don't sup-pose it works for everyone, but it has worked for me.

So, I will continue seeing Michael, continue working at my new relationship with Melanie – and my new relationship with my mother. I have yet to talk to Barry or Lucy, but I imagine that it will mark another significant step when I do, perhaps for all of us. I'm already thinking of visiting Lucy in Australia, and taking Melanie with me. I'd like them to meet. Lucy was there for me a lot as a child. I can feel myself becoming quite emotional as I realise that it is probably more impor-tant for me that Melanie gets on well with Lucy as compared to my mother. But we shall see. I feel inwardly – and outwardly – uncaged. I can feel beauty in my heart. I feel loved and I am learning to love. I have a future that I can walk towards with a smile.

Michael reflects on his experience as Peter's counsellor

You never know what to expect with a new client. I guess I was surprised at just how much happened over a relatively short space of time. It's not that it is unusual, it does happen, and I have seen change over a much shorter period. It often seems to depend on where the client is in their own process of change when they enter into therapy. It feels to me that Peter was ready for it, even though he probably didn't really know what he was letting himself in for.

I really felt I warmed to him and, yes, he did leave me with lots of feelings – both towards him and towards his mother. I felt like I was connected with him for much of the time. There were difficult, uncomfortable encounters, but that's how it can be sometimes.

Looking at Peter now I find myself wanting to smile. He has a life. He has got so many more possibilities open to him. Of course they were always there, but he wasn't in a position to see them, or maybe want them enough. He has created opportunities for himself and made good use of them. He has found a set of experiences that are more satisfying and he has sought to make them a more permanent feature in his life.

I don't know how many more sessions we will have. I don't need to know. Peter will know when it is helpful, and when it feels right to withdraw. I trust that. I also trust that I will sense this as well. No point in pre-planning anything. I'll go with it, keep offering Peter the empathic understanding, unconditional positive regard and congruence that I firmly believe to have such therapeutic value.

Of course, Peter's process of change has extended beyond the therapy room, both in terms of cause and effect. That feels good. It feels balanced. He's experiencing a life beyond the counselling room. Not all clients feel that way. Some become highly dependent on the counselling relationship, or live a life that is centred on that therapeutic experience. That is OK as well if that is what they need, if that is what brings them the kind of satisfying and self-validating experience that they need to feel more present as a person.

As I think back over the sessions I kind of have this sense of the actualising tendency seeking an outlet, seeking to find expression through the subtle shifts that occurred for Peter. 'Moving on' was such a powerful theme for him, and yet at the start he had no idea what to move on to, or how it would work out. In fact, it was more a case of an urge to 'get away' than to 'move on' – a very different emphasis. The drive to get away from something might not be seen as so positive as the urge to move on. Perhaps Peter moved from wanting to end something to an attitude of wanting to begin something new. After all, endings are also beginnings, it depends on your point of view. Peter has a lot of beginnings in his life. He has let light into his life, into his relationship with his mother. I know he didn't think it was courageous. But I still do. And I smile as I think about it.

Yes, it takes a determination to break free of a pattern that has been established from formative years. It is a step into the unknown, and that takes courage in my book. I have no doubt that the satisfaction that emerged within himself, and the shift in his self-concept that was associated with this – as someone who could love and feel loved – provided a powerful focus for the actualising tendency. And all the time he was embracing and reinforcing this fresh sense of self through his developing relationship with Melanie.

What part did I play? I listened. I offered him warmth, and I hope a consistent and accepting presence. I tried to be open and real, to be in touch with myself while I offered therapeutic relationship. I think I was generally responsive and appropriate. There were difficult times, and yet they seemed to lead to learning and insight. For me it is about how I am with clients more than what I do. I hope I have been, and will continue to be, a companion for Peter on his journey into himself. I feel good, I feel optimistic and I very much look forward to our future sessions and to sharing in his process of being able to not only acknowledge and accept that part of him who will perhaps always be his mother's son, but also develop a clearer presence of Peter the man, able to confidently relate not only to his mother, but also to Melanie as an adult. I hope that he will internalise more deeply the reality of being lovable, unravelling and dispersing the 'conditions of worth' and introjected meanings that he attributed to himself in the past. Yes, I hope that through the process of therapy a positive difference will occur. I can't make the difference and I can't know what form that difference will take, but as a person-centred counsellor I can offer the facilitative relational experience that will offer opportunity for Peter to realise himself as a fuller, more complete, and more congruent, human being.

Epilogue

It has been an enjoyable book to write. This may seem a strange statement to make, but I have watched and felt Peter change as the story unfolded. I started with a young man seeking help. As I wrote his first words, 'Er, hallo', I had no idea what would occur in the counselling sessions that followed. Yet I had a sense throughout that Peter would find a way of moving on although the triggers for this were at the start unknown to me, indeed, they remained unknown until they emerged into the dialogue during the process of writing.

Michael, his counsellor, was clearly affected by Peter. Michael is gay but I did not expand on this in the book, or make an issue out of it. So Michael is a gay man who happens to be a counsellor. Should I have had him exploring in supervision his physical contact with his male client? I thought about this after having completed the book, but was glad that I had not. It wasn't an issue. As I wrote the sessions where there was physical contact I had no sense that there was anything other than a fellow human being responding to another human being in pain. That was how I sensed the process and therefore that was what took form in the dialogue.

It is always a strange sensation ending a *Living Therapy* book. I am always left with a sense of wanting to know what comes next, as if I should write a few more pages to reveal – perhaps as much to myself as to the reader – how Peter's life shapes up in the future. He will carry sensitivities with him, no doubt, and I was pleased that there was a reconciliation with his mother. I know that this does not always occur, and the desperate search for approval and love can remain a driving urge in the son for the rest of their lives. Perhaps now Peter will experience greater acceptance from his mother, and maybe he will begin to know something of the love that he never experienced as a child. Peter struggled with the meaning of love, of what it meant to him, of how he would recognise it. Love. Such a small word and yet, perhaps, the greatest mystery of life. Love draws us on, moves us, takes us on journeys into ourselves.

What about daughters and mothers? Yes, they too can have problematic relationships that can lead to similar experiences. I have worked with women who, in adulthood, are still struggling to free themselves from their mothers, a condition often exacerbated later in life when a daughter may take on a caring role, still driven to find love and approval yet also experiencing anger and frustration, and then guilt in response to their anger.

Human beings are relational beings, even when we choose to be on our own, we are likely to be thinking or feeling about something – relating to experiences within ourselves. I hope that this book leaves you, the reader, with a sense of hope in the potential of human beings to grow out of difficult and negative experiences. Not everyone achieves this, of course. For some it is too much and they turn to a self-destructive lifestyle, perhaps involving alcohol, drugs or other addictive behaviours as they try to destroy the awfulness that fills their being and in so doing destroy themselves. But many do grow, move on, discover new potentialities and enriching experiences. Peter found Michael at a time in his life when he was beginning to realise something had to happen, something had to change. He found Melanie, he found music helping him connect with his drive to make changes, and he found, in *Phantom of the Opera*, someone that spoke to him at a deep and meaningful level. He moved on.

I am glad I wrote this book. It is shorter than some of the others in the series, something I had not appreciated until I received the page proofs. At first it troubled me – would readers feel short-changed? But then, to have extended it would have been simply to have done so for no reason other than to add words. For me, the therapeutic process had reached a point at which it felt right to end the narrative, even though the sessions would continue. Of course, a lot happened in those twelve sessions, and some might suggest that it was unrealistic within this time-frame. Yet I have seen clients change dramatically in much shorter periods of therapy, and I have seen people need to work for much longer to establish the trust they need in order for them to feel able to make visible aspects of their nature that had previously remained hidden.

I hope the characters in this book have touched you. We are all affected, to some greater or lesser extent, by our past experiences and the way we internalised them and shaped our self-concept. More and more people it seems are today seeking paths that enable them to challenge themselves, offering opportunity to break free from the patterns from their past that have become chains in the present. It was some years ago at a Conference that I heard a speaker say: '*the real pioneers in therapy are not those who formulate new theories, we have all the theories we need. The real pioneers are the clients*'. It is our clients who teach us so much about the complexity and the process of being human, the wonder and the despair, the love and the pain. The counsellor is privileged to share their journey with them.

References

Bozarth J (1998) *Person-Centred Therapy: a revolutionary paradigm*. PCCS Books, Ross-on-Wye.

Bozarth J and Wilkins P (eds) (2001) *Rogers' Therapeutic Conditions: evolution, theory and practice*. Volume 3: *Unconditional positive regard*. PCCS Books, Ross-on-Wye.

Bryant-Jefferies R (2003a) *Counselling a Recovering Drug User: a person-centred dialogue*. Radcliffe Medical Press, Oxford.

Bryant-Jefferies R (2003b) *Counselling Young People: person-centred dialogues*. Radcliffe Medical Press, Oxford.

Bryant-Jefferies R (2004) *Counselling for Progressive Disability: person-centred dialogues*. Radcliffe Medical Press, Oxford.

Gaylin N (2001) *Family, Self and Psychotherapy: a person-centred perspective*. PCCS Books, Ross-on-Wye.

Haugh S and Merry T (eds) (2001) *Rogers' Therapeutic Conditions: evolution, theory and practice*: Volume 2: *Empathy*. PCCS Books, Ross-on-Wye.

Mearns D (2000) The nature of 'configurations' within self. In: D Mearns and B Thorne (eds) *Person-Centred Therapy Today*. Sage Publications, London.

Mearns D and Thorne B (1988) *Person-Centred Counselling in Action*. Sage, London.

Mearns D and Thorne B (1999) *Person-Centred Counselling in Action* (2e). Sage, London.

Mearns D and Thorne B (2000) *Person-Centred Therapy Today*. Sage Publications, London.

Merry T (2002) *Learning and Being in Person-Centred Counselling* (2e). PCCS Books, Ross-on-Wye.

Patterson CH (2000) *Understanding Psychotherapy: fifty years of client-centred theory and practice*. PCCS Books, Ross-on-Wye.

Rogers CR (1942) *Counselling and Psychotherapy: newer concepts in practice*. Houghton Mifflin, Boston, MA.

Rogers CR (1957) The necessary and sufficient conditions of therapeutic personality change. *Journal of Consulting Psychology*. **21**: 95–103.

Rogers CR (1959) A theory of therapy, personality and interpersonal relationships as developed in the client-centred framework. In: S Koch (ed.) *Psychology: a study of a science*. Volume 3: *Formulations of the person and the social context*. McGraw-Hill, New York, pp. 219–35.

Rogers CR (1980) *A Way of Being.* Houghton Mifflin, Boston, MA.

Rogers CR (1986) A client-centered/person-centered approach to therapy. In: I Kutash and A Wolfe (eds) *Psychotherapists' Casebook.* Jossey-Bass, San Francisco, pp. 236–57.

Steinman J (1993) *Bat Out of Hell.* Carlin Music Corp.

Thorne B (1996) Person-centred therapy. In: W Dryden (ed.) *Handbook of Individual Therapy.* Sage, London.

Warner M (2002) Psychological contact, meaningful process and human nature. In: G Wyatt and P Sanders (eds) *Rogers' Therapeutic Conditions: evolution, theory and practice.* Volume 4: *Contact and perception.* PCCS Books, Ross-on-Wye, pp. 76–95.

Wilkins P (2003) *Person Centred Therapy in Focus.* Sage, London.

Wyatt G (ed.) (2001) *Rogers' Therapeutic Conditions: evolution, theory and practice.* Volume 1: *Congruence.* PCCS Books, Ross-on-Wye.

Wyatt G and Sanders P (eds) (2002) *Rogers' Therapeutic Conditions: evolution, theory and practice.* Volume 4: *Contact and perception.* PCCS Books, Ross-on-Wye.

Useful contacts

Person-centred

Association for the Development of the Person-Centered Approach (ADPCA)
Email: adpca-web@signs.portents.com
Website: www.adpca.org

An international association, with members in 27 countries, for those interested in the development of client-centred therapy and the person-centred approach.

British Association for the Person-Centred Approach (BAPCA)
Bm-BAPCA
London WC1N 3XX
Tel: 01989 770948
Email: info@bapca.org.uk
Website: www.bapca.org.uk

National association promoting the person-centred approach. Publishes the journal *Person-Centred Practice* and a regular newsletter *Person-to-Person*.

Person Centred Therapy Scotland
Tel: 0870 7650871
Email: info@pctscotland.co.uk
Website: www.pctscotland.co.uk

An association of person-centred therapists in Scotland which offers training and networking opportunities to members, with the aim of fostering high standards of professional practice.

World Association for Person-Centered and Experiential Psychotherapy and Counselling
Email: secretariat@pce-world.org
Website: www.pce-world.org

Index